Managing Cholesterol

by Simon Poole, MD, and Amy Riolo

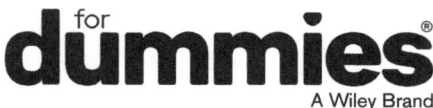

for
dummies®
A Wiley Brand

Managing Cholesterol For Dummies®

Published by: **John Wiley & Sons, Inc.**, 111 River Street, Hoboken, NJ 07030-5774, www.wiley.com

For general information on our other products and services, please contact our Customer Care Department within the U.S. at 877-762-2974, outside the U.S. at 317-572-3993, or fax 317-572-4002. For technical support, please visit https://hub.wiley.com/community/support/dummies.

Wiley publishes in a variety of print and electronic formats and by print-on-demand. Some material included with standard print versions of this book may not be included in e-books or in print-on-demand. If this book refers to media that is not included in the version you purchased, you may download this material at http://booksupport.wiley.com. For more information about Wiley products, visit www.wiley.com.

Library of Congress Control Number: 2025944155

ISBN 978-1-394-33106-2 (pbk); ISBN 978-1-394-33108-6 (ebk); ISBN 978-1-394-33107-9 (ebk)

Printed and bound by CPI Group (UK) Ltd, Croydon, CR0 4YY

C9781394331062_180825

Contents at a Glance

Introduction 1

Part 1: Understanding Cholesterol 5

CHAPTER 1: Why Cholesterol Matters for Health 7

CHAPTER 2: Defining Cholesterol. 17

CHAPTER 3: Understanding High Cholesterol 29

CHAPTER 4: Appreciating Oxidative Stress and Inflammation 39

Part 2: Changing Your Diet to Manage Cholesterol 59

CHAPTER 5: Understanding the Role of Cholesterol and the Diet 61

CHAPTER 6: Discovering the Best Diet for Cholesterol Management 79

Part 3: Assessing Risks 97

CHAPTER 7: Calculating the Risk of Cholesterol 99

CHAPTER 8: Understanding Your Individual Risk 109

CHAPTER 9: Reducing Risk through Self-Care, Sleep, and Connection 123

CHAPTER 10: Reducing Risk through Exercise and Stress Management 133

Part 4: Incorporating Medicines and Holistic Approaches 147

CHAPTER 11: Evaluating Treatment Options for Cholesterol 149

CHAPTER 12: Choosing a Holistic Approach. 165

Part 5: Heading into the Kitchen 173

CHAPTER 13: Cooking and Eating to Manage Cholesterol. 175

CHAPTER 14: Organizing the Kitchen and Meals. 195

CHAPTER 15: Recipes 211

Part 6: The Part of Tens 249

CHAPTER 16: Ten Easy Wins to Manage Cholesterol 251

CHAPTER 17: Ten Cholesterol-Friendly Foods to Incorporate into Your Diet. 259

CHAPTER 18: Ten Misconceptions about Cholesterol 267

Index 275

Recipes at a Glance

Base Recipes

Baby Artichokes 190
Cannellini Beans 188
Dried Beans 186
Dried Chickpeas 187
Fresh Breadcrumbs 193
Homemade Chicken Stock 185
Homemade Vegetable Stock 184
Lentils 189
Roasted Red Peppers 192
Tomato Basil Sauce 183
Za'atar Spiced Pita Chips 191

Breakfast

Apple Cinnamon Oatmeal with Toasted Almonds 216
Chocolate Ginger Waffles with Vanilla Berry Syrup 220
Greek Yogurt with Honey, Pomegranate, and Avocado Parfait 218
Red Berry, Dark Chocolate, and Chia Seed Overnight Pudding 217
Sweet Cardamom-Scented Barley and Strawberry Pudding with Nuts 219

Appetizers

Classic Hummus with Crudites 227
Pomegranate and Walnut Dip with Za'atar Spiced Pita Chips 222
Red Lentil "Meatballs" with Tomato Basil Sauce 225
Spiced Quinoa and Lentil Sliders 223

Soups and Salads

Artichoke, Pea, and Cherry Tomato Salad with Lemon and Basil Dressing 237
Avocado, Citrus, and Spinach Salad with Walnuts and White Balsamic
    Vinaigrette 240
Italian Barley, Bean, and Mixed Vegetable Soup 224
Moroccan Carrot Salad 239
Red Cabbage, Citrus, and Carrot Slaw with Cilantro Vinaigrette 236
Spinach, Lentil, and Pomegranate Salad 238

Main Courses

℧ Barley and Red Wine "Risotto" with Red Cabbage and Cannellini Beans. 233

Herb-Roasted "Plaki"-Style Fish with Vegetables and Brown Rice Pilaf 230

℧ Italian Pasta with Creamy Lentils and Pecorino Cheese 234

Marinated Salmon and Brussels Sprouts over Citrus Cream Sauce 229

℧ Vegetable Stir-Fry with Edamame and Brown Rice Noodles 232

Desserts

℧ Decadent Dark Chocolate Mousse with Strawberries. 246

℧ Fresh Summer Berry Clafoutis. 247

℧ Individual Spiced Apple Pies with Almond and Oatmeal Crust 242

℧ Italian Grape Harvest Cake with Cinnamon–Red Wine Reduction 244

℧ Orange and Olive Oil Walnut Cake 248

Table of Contents

INTRODUCTION 1
About This Book... 1
Foolish Assumptions... 2
Icons Used in This Book 2
Beyond the Book.. 3
Where to Go from Here 3

PART 1: UNDERSTANDING CHOLESTEROL 5

CHAPTER 1: **Why Cholesterol Matters for Health** 7
What Cholesterol Means for You 8
What Causes Heart Disease.. 9
How Cardiovascular Diseases Harm the Body 11
Why an Integrated Approach Counts................................. 13
  Preventing or treating disease by managing risk 13
  Modifying lifestyle and drawing on culinary medicine........... 15

CHAPTER 2: **Defining Cholesterol** 17
Recognizing the Importance of Cholesterol 17
  Appreciating the role of cholesterol in the body 18
  Identifying the types of circulating cholesterol................. 19
Measuring Cholesterol 21
  Interpreting the results.. 22
  Paying attention to your cholesterol ratio......................... 25
Beyond the Basics: Looking at Additional Tests 26

CHAPTER 3: **Understanding High Cholesterol**................... 29
Familial High Cholesterol: Blame It on Genetics.................. 30
Other Causes of High Cholesterol.................................... 31
  Diet 32
  Lack of physical activity.. 32
  Obesity 33
  Type 2 diabetes 33
  Chronic kidney or liver disease 33
  Long-term alcohol use 34
  Chronic stress and poor sleep....................................... 34
  Smoking and air pollution 35
  Medications 35
  Hormonal imbalances.. 35
  Chronic inflammatory states 36
  Life stages: Aging, pregnancy, and menopause 37

CHAPTER 4: **Appreciating Oxidative Stress and Inflammation**. 39

Looking at the Lipid Theory of Cholesterol and Chronic Disease 40
Understanding the lipid theory. 41
Understanding how cholesterol leads to chronic disease. 45
Measuring the effects of cholesterol 46
Focusing on Oxidation and Inflammation 47
Oxidized cholesterol. 48
Oxidative stress 49
Inflammation 51
Identifying the Diseases Caused by High Cholesterol 53
Heart attack 54
Stroke 55
Other vascular diseases 56
The special case of diabetes 56

PART 2: CHANGING YOUR DIET TO MANAGE CHOLESTEROL. 59

CHAPTER 5: **Understanding the Role of Cholesterol and the Diet** 61

Identifying Foods That Raise Cholesterol. 62
Trans fats 62
Saturated fats. 63
Refined carbohydrates 65
Excess alcohol 65
Processed foods 65
Foods that increase oxidative stress and inflammation 67
Foods cooked at high temperatures. 67
Excess salt. 68
Focusing on Cholesterol-Friendly Foods 71
Recognizing the importance of fiber 71
Appreciating healthy fats and stanols 73
Powering up with protein. 74
Getting the right vitamins and minerals 74
Managing oxidative stress with polyphenols 75
Grasping the role of the gut microbiome 76

CHAPTER 6: **Discovering the Best Diet for Cholesterol Management** 79

Defining the Mediterranean Diet 80
Comparing the Mediterranean Diet to the Western Diet 82
Weighing the Evidence for the Mediterranean Diet. 85

Making the Mediterranean Diet Work for You .87
    Incorporating the foods that lower cholesterol 87
    Reducing oxidative stress and inflammation 91

PART 3: ASSESSING RISKS. 97

CHAPTER 7: Calculating the Risk of Cholesterol. 99
Understanding the Difference between Primary
Prevention and Secondary Prevention. 99
    Considering levels of risk in primary prevention 101
    Treating for risk reduction 102
Making Sense of Risk Assessment Tools 105
    The ASCVD Risk Estimator 105
    The QRISK Risk Calculator 106
    Other algorithms 106

CHAPTER 8: Understanding Your Individual Risk 109
Interpreting the Risks 110
    Knowing what a risk score means for you. 110
    Recognizing the limitations of risk tools 111
Working with Your Doctor to Treat (or Not Treat)
Your Cholesterol 114
    Knowing when to start or stop statins .115
    Talking with your doctor about treatment. 118

**CHAPTER 9: Reducing Risk through Self-Care, Sleep,
and Connection** 123
Taking Time for Self-Care. 124
Getting Good-Quality Sleep 126
    Seeing how sleep helps regulate cholesterol 126
    Improving your sleep 127
Keeping Connected. 129
    Understanding how connection helps .129
    Creating and maintaining connection .130

**CHAPTER 10: Reducing Risk through Exercise and Stress
Management** 133
Enjoying Exercise. 134
    Recognizing the benefits of exercise 134
    Choosing the exercise that's right for you 136
Reducing Stress 137
    Seeing how stress affects cholesterol and
    cardiovascular risk. 139
    Managing stress. 140

PART 4: INCORPORATING MEDICINES AND
HOLISTIC APPROACHES 147

CHAPTER 11: **Evaluating Treatment Options for Cholesterol** ... 149

Knowing When Medications Are Considered for High
Cholesterol 150
Secondary prevention 150
Primary prevention 152
Surveying the Medications Used to Treat High Cholesterol 153
Statins 154
Cholesterol absorption inhibitors 154
Bile acid sequestrants 155
Fibrates 155
Niacin 155
PCSK9 inhibitors 156
MTP inhibitors 156
ACL inhibitors 156
Omega-3 fatty acids 157
Personalizing Therapy 157
Considering targets and dosing 158
Knowing how low to go 159
Watching for drug interactions 160
Monitoring treatment and side effects 161
Looking at Other Common Treatments for Cardiovascular
Disease 162
Surgical interventions 162
Other common treatments for CVD 163

CHAPTER 12: **Choosing a Holistic Approach** 165

Holistic Approaches 165
Complementary Therapies 167
Acupuncture 168
Emotional Freedom Technique (also known as tapping) 169
Reiki 169
Supplements 170
Metaphysical healing 170

PART 5: HEADING INTO THE KITCHEN 173

CHAPTER 13: **Cooking and Eating to Manage Cholesterol** 175

Cooking to Manage Cholesterol 175
Planning meals 176
Cooking with antioxidant-rich foods 177
Avoiding unhealthful fats 179
Making Whole Foods Taste Great 180
Preparing Base Recipes 182

CHAPTER 14: **Organizing the Kitchen and Meals** 195

Organizing Your Kitchen 195
    Setting yourself up for success 196
    Stocking your pantry 197
    Filling the freezer 198
    Focusing on the fridge 199
Finding Time to Cook 199
Planning Meals 201
    Setting a schedule that works for you 202
    Looking at a sample seven-day meal plan 203
Eating Out with Pleasure and Health in Mind 208

CHAPTER 15: **Recipes** 211

Finding Cholesterol-Friendly Foods 212
Breakfast 214
Savory Appetizers and Small Plates 221
Hearty Main Courses 228
Satisfying Salads 235
Dazzling Desserts 241

PART 6: THE PART OF TENS 249

CHAPTER 16: **Ten Easy Wins to Manage Cholesterol** 251

Increasing Your Fiber Intake 251
Choosing Healthy Fats 252
Reading Food Labels 253
Focusing on a Sustainable Mediterranean Diet 253
Embracing Extra-Virgin Olive Oil 254
Planning Your Meals 255
Enjoying More Exercise 255
Sleeping Well 256
Taking Care of Yourself 256
Checking Out Other Risks for Cardiovascular Disease 257

CHAPTER 17: **Ten Cholesterol-Friendly Foods to Incorporate into Your Diet** 259

Herbs and Spices 260
Beans and Other Legumes 261
Nuts and Seeds 261
Extra-Virgin Olive Oil 263
Fish 263
Whole Grains 264
Greek Yogurt 264
Fruits and Vegetables 265

CHAPTER 18: **Ten Misconceptions about Cholesterol**............267

Myth: All Cholesterol Is Bad...................................267

Myth: Cholesterol Is the Most Important Risk Factor..............268

Myth: Only Overweight People Have High Cholesterol...........269

Myth: Cholesterol Simply Blocks Arteries 269

Myth: Everything That Matters Is Measured in Risk
Calculator Tools...270

Myth: Success Is Measured by a Lipid Panel....................270

Myth: You Can't Lower Cholesterol Risk without Medications......271

Myth: I Can Eat Whatever I Want Because I Take a Statin.........272

Myth: A Low-Fat Diet Is Best 273

Myth: Sugar Has No Effect on Cholesterol.....................273

INDEX..275

Introduction

You may be reading this book because you've had your cholesterol measured or perhaps because a friend or relative has been told that they have high cholesterol.

Maybe you're confused about what cholesterol actually is, what causes it to rise, what the numbers mean, and how this may affect your health. You probably also want to know how you can have better conversations with your doctor about the implications of test results and, most important, how you can manage your cholesterol.

You'll be delighted to hear that the advice contained in this book combines the most up-to-date, evidence-based medical knowledge with a truly holistic approach to achieve the best diet and lifestyle for your cholesterol and general health and well-being.

About This Book

This book demystifies cholesterol and provides effective solutions for preventing high cholesterol, managing existing cholesterol levels, and achieving a lower cholesterol overall. This new, holistic, and integrative approach to cholesterol management offers real hope for people looking not only to lower their cholesterol numbers, but also to avoid the complications that are associated with higher cholesterol in the first place. It explains the best way to manage the risks of cardiovascular disease (CVD), including heart attacks and strokes, which are associated with a high cholesterol.

You can find more information about specific conditions such as heart disease in *Preventing & Reversing Heart Disease For Dummies* by James Rippe (John Wiley & Sons). There is a deeper dive into the dietary and lifestyle approach introduced in this book in titles such as *Mediterranean Lifestyle For Dummies* by Amy Riolo and *Olive Oil For Dummies* by Amy Riolo and Simon Poole, MD (both published by John Wiley & Sons).

Managing Cholesterol For Dummies explains the evolution of the latest scientific knowledge and helps you understand the best ways to handle your cholesterol through lifestyle changes, medical treatments, and other therapies. The easy and mouthwatering recipes in Chapter 15 focus not only on the important ingredients known to reduce "bad" cholesterol but also on the delicious antioxidant-rich foods that decrease the oxidation of cholesterol and control inflammation for optimal cholesterol management.

Within this book, you may note that some web addresses break across two lines of text. If you're reading this book in print and want to visit one of these web pages, simply key in the web address exactly as it's noted in the text, pretending as though the line break doesn't exist. If you're reading this as an e-book, you've got it easy — just click the web address to be taken directly to the web page.

Foolish Assumptions

In writing this book, we made a few assumptions about you, our reader:

>> You don't know very much about cholesterol, but you may have heard that a high cholesterol level can affect your health.

>> You aren't already familiar with all the ingredients that can be used to raise "good" cholesterol and lower "bad" cholesterol, as well as those with anti-inflammatory effects.

>> You don't know how to prepare the types of meals that someone managing cholesterol should prepare.

>> You're curious and interested and willing to try new things — especially if it means improving your quality of life.

Icons Used in This Book

The icons in the margins of this book point out information we think is especially important. Here are the icons used in this book:

REMEMBER

Remember icons mark the information that's especially important to know. To siphon off the most important information in each chapter, just skim through these icons.

TIP

The Tip icon marks important information that can save you time and energy.

WARNING

Watch for the Warning icon — it warns about potential problems (for example, the possible results if you don't treat a condition).

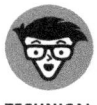

TECHNICAL STUFF

The Technical Stuff icon marks information of a highly technical nature that you can normally skip over.

Beyond the Book

In addition to the material in the print or e-book you're reading right now, this product also comes with some access-anywhere goodies on the web. Check out this book's online Cheat Sheet. Just go to www.dummies.com and type **Managing Cholesterol For Dummies Cheat Sheet** in the Search box. You'll find tips on quick and easy ways to achieve your cholesterol goals.

Where to Go from Here

Where you go from here depends on your immediate needs. If you're looking for something to make for dinner tonight, head to Chapter 15. If you've just gotten your lipid panel results and you're trying to make sense of all those numbers, head to Chapter 3. If you're wanting to understand more about the best diet for cholesterol management, turn to Chapter 6, or if you need to learn more about medications, turn to Chapter 11. And if you're not sure where to turn, you can start reading Chapter 1 — or use the Table of Contents or Index to find the information that most interests you.

Many of the changes we suggest can take some time to implement. The good news is that they involve positive, enjoyable, and sustainable transitions that have much broader beneficial effects than simply reducing your cholesterol.

1

Understanding Cholesterol

IN THIS PART . . .

Make a whole-person approach to cholesterol management work.

Understand why cholesterol matters in health.

Witness how the story of cholesterol has changed.

Appreciate how oxidation and inflammation affect cholesterol and why tackling them is key to protecting your heart.

See how lifestyle and culinary medicine can help.

Chapter **1**

Why Cholesterol Matters for Health

Odds are, you hear a lot about cholesterol. It's one of the most common blood tests recommended by doctors and requested by patients — about two-thirds of U.S. adults say they've had their cholesterol checked within the last five years. According to the World Health Organization (WHO), approximately 40 percent of adults worldwide have high cholesterol. In 2024, the U.S. Centers for Disease Control and Prevention (CDC) estimated that 86 million adults in the United States have cholesterol levels that are considered borderline or high. In 2024, the value of cholesterol-lowering medications produced by the pharmaceutical industry was $34 billion and it's predicted to rise to $50 billion by 2033.

But what does this mean for you? To answer that question, you need to know the role of cholesterol in the body, the risks associated with high cholesterol, the latest research that's changing our understanding of the link between cholesterol and disease, and the role of lifestyle and medications in keeping our cholesterol levels and blood vessels healthy.

In this chapter, you begin to appreciate the importance of cholesterol and why it's appropriate to ask questions and perhaps challenge some of the previous assumptions about how best to manage your results. Many people feel disempowered by a lack of understanding of the risks of high cholesterol and the pros and cons of taking medication. With the help of the different approach of this book, you can take back that control!

What Cholesterol Means for You

If you've had your cholesterol measured, it was probably done in the form of a *full lipid panel* or *full lipid profile,* which is a test of circulating fats that include different types of cholesterol. (We describe the elements that make up this complete result and their significance in Chapter 2.)

You may have requested a blood test because you heard it's important to know your cholesterol level, or your doctor may have ordered the blood test as part of an annual checkup or possibly because you have symptoms of an illness, whether associated with cholesterol or not.

The importance of knowing your cholesterol level stems from the association of high levels of some types of circulating cholesterol with *vascular pathology* (a disease of the blood vessels that can lead to many different illnesses, including the most common causes of death and sickness in most countries — heart disease and stroke).

But there is much more to the story of cholesterol and the risk of heart disease and stroke than first meets the eye. There is certainly more than is known to many physicians and much more than can be explained in a brief consultation, which may result in a patient committing to lifelong medication. Many aspects of cholesterol remain poorly understood. Not everyone with high cholesterol will end up getting sick. Given that cholesterol levels can vary along a spectrum, the definition of a high cholesterol is inevitably somewhat arbitrary. Plus, there is debate about what causes high cholesterol for many people, as well as controversy about the extent to which highly effective cholesterol medications may cause significant side effects.

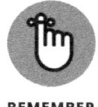

REMEMBER

During 35 years of clinical practice as a physician in primary care, Simon has had countless consultations with patients about cholesterol — discussing blood tests, risk assessment, and possible treatment for high cholesterol. The challenge for all doctors is to provide enough accurate and up-to-date information within the constraints of the time available, so every patient is in a position to make a fully informed and individual decision about what's best for them and how to consider if those judgments may change over time.

What Causes Heart Disease

All parts of the body — whether it's the heart, brain, muscles, lungs, kidneys, or any other organ — depend on a healthy blood supply to fulfill their various functions. The blood vessels that supply oxygen, nutrients, immune support, and hormones to effectively sustain the cells that perform the tasks for life are called *arteries.* Together with *veins,* which take the blood back to the heart, they're collectively described as the *vascular system.*

TECHNICAL STUFF

Larger blood vessels, which carry blood over longer distances, are part of the *macrovascular system.* Branches of blood vessels get smaller as they approach the cells they support; here, the arteries become *arterioles* and *capillaries* and are described as the *microvascular system.*

Arteriosclerosis is a condition in which the arteries are hardened and thickened, with fatty or calcified deposits known as *plaques.* A similar term, *atherosclerosis,* is more specifically used when describing plaques in larger arteries. (See the nearby sidebar for more on the coining of this term and the study of heart disease over the past couple hundred years.) The changes visible in blood vessels affected by atherosclerosis are shown in Figure 1-1.

FIGURE 1-1:
A blood vessel showing signs of developing changes of atherosclerosis.

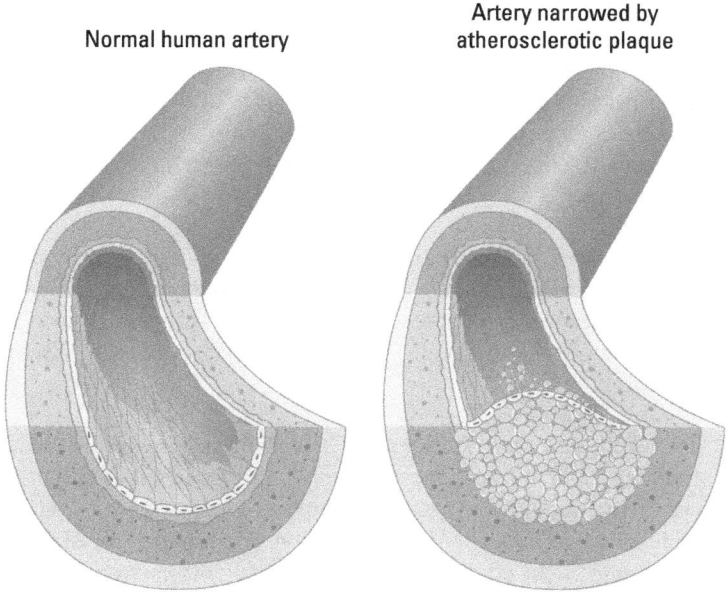

Normal human artery

Artery narrowed by atherosclerotic plaque

© *John Wiley & Sons, Inc.*

So, what does cholesterol have to do with it? Years ago, doctors believed that cholesterol (and saturated fat, which leads to cholesterol production) in the diet caused excess circulating fats, or *lipids,* and those excess lipids were deposited in blood vessel walls as plaques. The result was damage to and narrowing of the blood vessels, and ultimately blockage of blood supply to vital organs like the heart and brain. But today we know that the process by which cholesterol may be associated with heart disease, stroke, or other organ damage is complex. And the consequences of this understanding are significant.

The path to heart disease or any other vascular disease must be dependent on other factors. After all, not everyone with high cholesterol will develop problems. Plus, because of the complexity of the multiple risk factors for atherosclerosis and how they interact, people with identical cholesterol profiles may well have very different likelihoods of developing disease. It's obvious that there must be something else (or many other things) going on.

But the story is even more complicated: Cholesterol in the diet doesn't actually contribute most to blood cholesterol levels, and different fats can have adverse or beneficial effects. Other factors — including carbohydrate metabolism, diabetes, obesity, physical inactivity, some medications, and smoking — can affect cholesterol levels as well.

TIP

There have been numerous recent advances in research into the formation, structure and chemistry of blood vessel plaques and it is now possible to explain much more about their relationship with circulating cholesterol. We offer an up-to-date description of how plaques in blood vessels develop, become unstable, and lead to disease in more detail in Chapters 5, 9, and 10. When you understand this subject, you have the opportunity to make actionable changes in the management of your cholesterol.

Perhaps the greatest change in approach has come from the appreciation that plaque progression occurs as a result of chronic inflammation, and that a process called *cholesterol oxidation* contributes to this process — a phenomenon that has its own underlying causes and can vary significantly between individuals and over time.

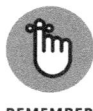

REMEMBER

Bottom line: The development of atherosclerosis is not just a matter of cholesterol. It relates to oxidation of cholesterol and inflammation of plaques, which can occur where there are excessive reactive oxygen atoms, described as *oxidative stress* and *chronic inflammation.* We explore this subject more extensively in Chapter 3. In addition, Chapters 4 and 10 focus on how you may be able to reduce that oxidation and inflammation with relatively easy changes to diet and lifestyle.

THE HISTORY OF THE STUDY OF HEART DISEASE: A CHANGING STORY

In the 17th and 18th centuries, anatomists began to explore the relationship between postmortem changes and diseases. In 1829, Jean Lobstein, a French pathologist, coined the term *arteriosclerosis*. Lobstein linked this condition to aging and disease, but the mechanism was unclear.

A few decades later, Rudolf Virchow, a German physician and scientist, proposed that plaques resulted from lipid accumulation and inflammation. He described how cholesterol deposits and cellular debris contributed to arterial blockage, forming the foundation for the modern understanding of atherosclerosis.

Early 20th-century researchers, including Nikolai Anichkov, demonstrated experimentally that dietary cholesterol could lead to arterial plaques in animals. This understanding solidified the connection between lipids, plaques, and vascular disease. By the mid-20th century, epidemiological studies, such as the Framingham Heart Study, connected high cholesterol levels and plaque buildup to cardiovascular events like heart attacks and strokes.

From the University of Washington, Seattle, Professor Russell Ross's 1999 article "Atherosclerosis — An Inflammatory Disease" in the *New England Journal of Medicine* was a landmark publication that redefined atherosclerosis as a chronic inflammatory condition. It emphasized the role of blood vessel wall injury from smoking and pollution toxins, chemical changes of high glucose or cholesterol levels, and the physical stress from high blood pressure as the initiating event, triggering an immune response, which promotes inflammation, leading to plaque buildup and arterial narrowing. Cholesterol trapped in the arterial wall can undergo a process called *oxidation* (damage from circulating reactive oxygen atoms), which triggers an immune response and makes this a central player in plaque formation and inflammation.

How Cardiovascular Diseases Harm the Body

The supply of blood through blood vessels to the organs is essential for the organs' proper functioning and the maintenance of health. It's what keeps you alive. Disruption and compromise of the efficient passage of oxygen and nutrients carried by blood cells through those vessels is responsible for the illnesses that cause the most sickness and death in the majority of populations — *cardiovascular diseases* (CVDs), which include *coronary heart disease* and *cerebrovascular disease*, more familiarly referred to as heart disease and stroke, respectively.

When large blood vessels are affected, it may result in sudden events of critical loss of blood supply to a large area of an organ, such as a *myocardial infarction* (heart attack) or a *cerebrovascular accident* (stroke) affecting the brain. When the smaller blood vessels are more involved, more gradual and smaller incremental damage may occur and result in slower deterioration in functioning, such as in heart failure or vascular dementia.

CVDs are the leading cause of death globally. In 2019, an estimated 17.9 million people died from CVDs, representing 32 percent of all global deaths. Of these deaths, 85 percent were due to heart attack and stroke. CVDs are the leading cause of death and disability in the WHO European Region. An estimated 4.2 million people in Europe died from CVDs in 2019, representing 42.5 percent of all deaths. This is the highest proportion of all the WHO regions. According to the WHO, the majority of these deaths are preventable.

The CDC describes heart disease as the leading cause of death for men, women, and people of most racial and ethnic groups in the United States, with one person dying every 33 seconds from CVD. In 2022, 702,880 people died from heart disease. The cost of CVD was estimated to be about $252.2 billion from 2019 to 2020.

REMEMBER

The heart and brain are the organs that are most vulnerable to vascular diseases, but deficiencies in blood supply to other parts of the body can result in damage to the following:

>> **Kidneys:** Vascular diseases can impair blood flow to the kidneys, leading to kidney damage and chronic kidney disease.

>> **Lungs:** Vascular diseases can affect the blood vessels in the lungs, leading to conditions like *pulmonary embolism* (blood clot in the lungs) and *pulmonary hypertension* (high blood pressure in the lungs).

>> **Liver:** Vascular diseases can reduce blood flow to the liver, leading to liver damage and dysfunction.

>> **Limbs:** Vascular diseases, particularly *peripheral artery disease,* can affect the blood vessels in the legs and arms, causing pain and numbness, and potentially leading to tissue damage and amputation.

>> **Eyes:** Vascular diseases can affect the blood vessels in the eyes, leading to conditions like *diabetic retinopathy* (damage to the retina of the eye from diabetes) and *age-related macular degeneration* (age-related damage to central vision).

TIP

Optimum management of cholesterol is not just a numbers game. A low cholesterol number shouldn't in itself be the target — the desired outcome is a healthy and fulfilled life, free from the burden of illness.

WARNING

An article in the journal *Life* in 2016 that considered how physicians can influence lifestyle changes in patients at risk of heart disease noted a phenomenon referred to as *statin complacency* or *risk compensation*. This idea is based on the notion that people taking medications such as statins to lower cholesterol may feel a false sense of security, believing the medication is sufficient to manage their cardiovascular risk and, therefore, maintain a poor diet, feel no need to exercise, or even continue to smoke! Fortunately, there are also research papers that contradict this concern, showing that most people who receive adequate explanations about cholesterol, medication, and lifestyle tend to adopt more healthy behaviors. We look at medical treatments for high cholesterol in Chapter 11.

With any level of cholesterol, oxidation and inflammation, which are now known to be crucial to the development of CVD, are also critical factors. Measuring oxidation and inflammation isn't as straightforward, though, and because doctors generally rely on simple numbers that only provide the proportions of lipids, virtually no attention is given to levels of oxidation and inflammation. As Albert Einstein said, "Not everything that counts can be counted, and not everything that can be counted counts." Despite being a less measurable and tangible aspect of cholesterol, what is happening to the cholesterol circulating in the body must be central to any discussion about its management.

Why an Integrated Approach Counts

CVD and other vascular diseases are linked not just to high cholesterol, but to a number of other aspects of life: smoking, high blood pressure, poor diet, obesity, diabetes, and physical inactivity. Being male increases the risk, though following menopause the risk is similar if not higher in females, as well as having a family history of CVD. Risk further rises with age. Conditions of chronic inflammation and oxidative stress also increase rates of CVD. Having high cholesterol is just one of many factors, and it shouldn't be looked at in isolation. That's why it's important to consider an integrated approach to managing cholesterol and reducing the risk of CVD.

Preventing or treating disease by managing risk

When you manage cholesterol, you're managing a risk factor for vascular disease. The fact that CVD and other disorders of blood vessels are so common makes it an important consideration, but as a single risk factor, a high cholesterol level should not be thought of in isolation. Any gains in reducing cholesterol should be seen in the context of all other risk factors. On its own, raised cholesterol is a poor predictor of whether someone is likely to develop CVD, but where it exists among other risks, it becomes much more significant. (We explore the concept of risk in detail in Chapters 7 and 8.)

TIP

There is a big difference in the effects of reducing cholesterol levels depending on whether a person is known to have already established vascular disease. *Primary prevention* targets people without CVD to prevent its development, while *secondary prevention* focuses on individuals with CVD or risk factors to reduce the risk of future events.

The 4S Study was a landmark clinical trial published in the prestigious *Lancet* journal in November 1994 looking at people who had CVD. It demonstrated a 30 percent reduction in overall mortality and a 28 percent reduction in the risk of coronary heart disease events in patients with coronary heart disease who were treated with simvastatin, a cholesterol-lowering and oxidation-reducing medication in a class of drugs called statins. This study demonstrated the importance of cholesterol management in secondary prevention. Statins have become the cornerstone of medical prevention of further strokes, heart attacks, or other complications in people who have been diagnosed with vascular diseases or who are at high risk.

TIP

The reduction in risk of further events in the secondary prevention of CVD with statin treatment is very impressive. However, comparable risk reductions can be seen when people adopt a Mediterranean diet, exercise regularly, and stop smoking, showing that lifestyle changes in conjunction with medical treatments can be very effective and that one should not be a substitute for the other.

Primary prevention of CVD may also involve medications like statins; however, the reduced risks and lower potential gains mean that different considerations apply. The significance of modestly elevated cholesterol in a young person with no other risk factors is much less important than the implications of the same level in someone who is older or who has other risks of vascular disease.

Whether a person has their cholesterol checked at all may depend on where they live and what attitudes they and their doctor have about cholesterol and risk. In some countries, the approach to screening is much more proactive and there is a lower threshold for active management, surveillance, and treatment. In regions where this more anticipatory attitude is common, public health bodies issue guidelines encouraging doctors to screen. Sometimes there are financial incentives for health practitioners to identify and treat patients with high cholesterol. For example, in some countries pharmaceutical companies are allowed to advertise or even sell medications directly to the public; in other countries, legislation prohibits or limits this activity. How often you have your cholesterol checked, if at all, at what age, and whether this results in medication depends to some degree on where you live.

This reality makes understanding the implications of cholesterol even more important. It empowers you to know when to request a test, how to respond to an invitation for screening, and how to decide, in discussion with your doctor, on the best treatment for you.

Modifying lifestyle and drawing on culinary medicine

The majority of healthcare professionals receive most of their training applying the *medical model of care* (the traditional approach to healthcare focused on diagnosing and treating diseases primarily through clinical interventions such as medications, surgeries, and other acute care measures). Under the medical model of care, there is a tendency to emphasize identifying and addressing specific diseases or conditions and treating symptoms or managing crises rather than preventing illnesses. Although this model is often effective for acute illnesses and emergencies, it sometimes overlooks broader lifestyle and social determinants of health, such as diet, exercise, and mental well-being.

Increasingly, there is a drive to take a more holistic approach with the practice of complementary and aligned principles of *lifestyle medicine,* which takes a proactive, prevention-oriented approach to health by addressing the root causes of chronic diseases through lifestyle changes. Lifestyle medicine is built on principles of maintaining health and considering the whole person, engaging individuals as active participants in their health journey (including their physical, mental, and emotional well-being), and encouraging sustainable modifications in areas such as the following:

>> Nutrition

>> Physical activity

>> Sleep

>> Stress management

>> Substance avoidance

>> Social connectedness

>> Relaxation

Various components of lifestyle medicine — such as exercising, eating a healthful diet, losing weight if necessary, using healthful cooking methods, and reducing stress through yoga, tai chi, and meditation — may also help you to keep your cholesterol levels under control. Chapter 12 discusses various alternative therapies to consider as well.

Culinary medicine is a new field of medicine that combines the art of cooking with evidence-based nutritional science to help people achieve better health through food. It focuses on the role of dietary habits in preventing, managing, and even reversing chronic diseases while emphasizing the enjoyment and cultural significance of eating. Culinary medicine bridges the gap between knowing what to eat (nutrition) and making it practical and enjoyable (culinary skills), empowering individuals to take control of their health through food. This field recognizes that food is not only medicine but also a source of joy, culture, and connection.

TIP

The best way to optimize taking care of your cholesterol is through lifestyle and culinary medicine, with effective medical management explored if you and your healthcare professional agree that it's necessary and appropriate.

Chapter **2**

Defining Cholesterol

M ost people think of cholesterol as a number — a test result. That number may cause concern (because high levels of cholesterol carry an increased risk of the most common causes of sickness and death: heart disease and stroke). Maybe the number is a regular topic of conversation between you and your doctor. And perhaps the number results in disappointment when the figure seems to fluctuate beyond your control.

But there's more to cholesterol than just a scary or apparently reassuring number. Cholesterol is made by the body and performs functions in cells throughout the body, but it has to be transported to and from those cells through blood vessels. Too much circulating cholesterol in certain forms is associated with damage to the blood vessels, which results in cardiovascular disease, but there some forms of cholesterol that counter this risk and are beneficial.

In this chapter, we explain the role of cholesterol, spell out which types of cholesterol are the "good" and "bad" types, how cholesterol is measured, and the meaning of those results.

Recognizing the Importance of Cholesterol

Cholesterol is an essential component of the human body. It is present in every cell and circulates in the bloodstream. Despite its reputation as something harmful, cholesterol is vital for numerous bodily functions.

Cholesterol is a *sterol*, a type of *lipid* (fat) molecule made up of carbon, hydrogen, and oxygen atoms. Its unique structure allows it to interact with fats and water, making it a crucial component in cells and other systems such as carrying messages essential for life.

Although we get some cholesterol directly from foods, 70 percent to 80 percent of the cholesterol in the bloodstream is manufactured by the body. The liver is the primary organ responsible for cholesterol production; it synthesizes cholesterol from fats, carbohydrates, and proteins. Even without dietary cholesterol, the liver can produce all the cholesterol needed to maintain health.

The body is a great regulator. Through feedback mechanisms, the body tries to keep cholesterol levels in a natural balance. When there is more cholesterol in the diet, the liver produces less; conversely when dietary intake decreases, the liver compensates by producing more cholesterol. Cholesterol levels can rise for a number of reasons, and it's not always possible for the body to maintain healthy regulation of cholesterol, risking damage to blood vessels that supply vital organs. When there are high levels of cholesterol in the blood, this is sometimes referred to as *hypercholesterolemia*.

Appreciating the role of cholesterol in the body

Cholesterol fulfills several essential functions contributing to health, including the following:

» **Cholesterol is a building block for cell membranes.** Cholesterol is incorporated into the walls of cells to maintain the structure and permeability of cells. Cholesterol allows important nutrients and chemical messages to pass in and out of cells, while ensuring the cells' integrity.

» **Cholesterol is a precursor for hormones.** Cholesterol is the starting material for the synthesis of steroid hormones, including sex hormones (such as estrogen and testosterone) and adrenal hormones (such as cortisol). *Hormones* are chemical messengers that stimulate specific cells to act in ways to support life.

» **Cholesterol helps in the production of bile acids.** Bile acids, derived from cholesterol, are substances produced in the liver and released into the gut to aid in breaking down dietary fats and absorbing fat-soluble vitamins (vitamins A, D, E, and K).

>> **Cholesterol helps with the synthesis of vitamin D.** Sunlight converts cholesterol in the skin into vitamin D, a nutrient crucial for calcium absorption and immune health.

Cholesterol is especially important for the brain. In fact, the brain is the most cholesterol-rich organ in the body — it contains about 20 percent of the body's total cholesterol. Cholesterol is critical in the formation and maintenance of *synapses* (the connections between neurons essential for learning, memory, and overall brain function). It also contributes to the selective permeability of the blood-brain barrier, protecting the brain from harmful substances in the blood, while allowing nutrients to pass through. Cholesterol is a component of *myelin* (the fatty sheath that insulates nerve fibers and ensures efficient signal transmission between nerve cells). It also helps regulate the release of *neurotransmitters* (chemicals that transmit signals between nerve cells).

Identifying the types of circulating cholesterol

Cholesterol can't dissolve in blood, so it's transported by *lipoproteins*, which are complexes of lipids and proteins designed to carry fats, including cholesterol, through the bloodstream. The protein component helps make the fat more soluble in blood and directs it to where it's needed in the body. The main types of lipoproteins are:

>> **Low-density lipoprotein (LDL):** Often called "bad" cholesterol, LDL cholesterol carries cholesterol to tissues but can contribute to plaque buildup in arteries if levels are too high.

LDL has two subtypes:

   • **Small, dense LDL particles** are smaller and denser than larger LDL particles. They're more prone to oxidation, which makes them more likely to contribute to plaque buildup in the arteries. Studies have shown that having a high proportion of small, dense LDL particles is associated with an increased risk of heart disease, even if your total LDL cholesterol level is within a normal range.

   • **Large, buoyant LDL particles** are larger and less dense than small, dense LDL particles. They're generally considered less *atherogenic* (less likely to cause plaque buildup).

>> **High-density lipoprotein (HDL):** Known as "good" cholesterol, HDL cholesterol helps remove excess cholesterol from the bloodstream and transports it back to the liver for disposal or recycling. Moderately, but not excessively, high HDL cholesterol is considered to reduce the risk of heart disease.

HDL has two subtypes:

- **Large, mature HDL particles** are larger and contain more cholesterol.
- **Small, dense HDL particles** are smaller and contain less cholesterol.

  Some studies suggest the small HDL particles may have strong protective effects, but the overall function of HDL — including antioxidant and anti-inflammatory properties — and not just particle size, determines its cardiovascular benefit.

>> **Intermediate-density lipoprotein (IDL):** Formed during the transition from VLDL to LDL, these lipoproteins are temporary carriers of cholesterol and triglycerides.

>> **Chylomicrons:** These are the largest lipoprotein and carry mainly *triglycerides* (a type of fat used for energy storage and metabolism). After meals, triglycerides are absorbed from food in the gut and transported by these lipoproteins to tissues for immediate energy or storage in fat cells for future use.

>> **Very low-density lipoprotein (VLDL):** These lipoproteins carry triglycerides and cholesterol from the liver to tissues. They're considered a precursor to LDL because when they've delivered the triglycerides, they become denser and more like LDL.

Lipoproteins also carry the vitamins A, D, E and K, which are fat soluble, so they "hitch a ride" with lipoproteins, which can carry fats in the blood to where they're needed.

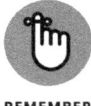

When cholesterol is being transported by lipoproteins through the circulatory system, especially in excess amounts, it's vulnerable to damaging chemical reactions, including *oxidation* (a process where unstable molecules called *free radicals* with unpaired electrons damage cells by stealing electrons from healthy molecules). Oxidized LDL can be retained in damaged blood vessel walls, forming plaques and triggering an immune response leading to the chronic inflammation that results in cardiovascular disease. We explain this process in more detail in Chapter 4.

The state of oxidation of LDL cholesterol is not measured, so it isn't possible to precisely understand how damaging any level of circulating cholesterol may be in practice. We discuss the limitations of cholesterol test results in more detail in the next section.

Measuring Cholesterol

A cholesterol blood test measures circulating cholesterol in the lipoproteins. The LDL cholesterol (LDL-C) component is associated with cardiovascular diseases, whereas the HDL cholesterol (HDL-C) gives protection. For this reason, it's difficult to interpret the meaning of a simple total cholesterol (TC) level. The TC may be made up of predominantly "bad" LDL-C or have a high level of "good" HDL-C. Without knowing the proportions of each component, it's not possible to say if a high TC level is a significant risk factor for cardiovascular disease and whether you should try to lower your levels.

A more accurate measurement is the *lipid panel test*, which provides levels of TC, LDL-C, and HDL-C. It may also include a measure of *non-HDL cholesterol*, which combines the levels of the LDL cholesterol and VLDL cholesterol. Other fats that are commonly measured in a lipid panel are circulating triglycerides (TGs), which we cover later in this chapter.

Here's a summary of the lipids most commonly measured in a lipid panel test:

>> **TC:** Measures the overall cholesterol level in your blood.

>> **LDL-C:** Often called "bad" cholesterol, high levels of LDL-C can increase the risk of plaque buildup in arteries, leading to heart disease or stroke.

>> **HDL-C:** Known as "good" cholesterol, HDL-C helps remove excess cholesterol from the bloodstream and transports it to the liver for excretion.

>> **TGs:** A type of fat in your blood. High levels are linked to an increased risk of heart disease, especially in combination with high LDL-C or low HDL-C.

>> **Non-HDL cholesterol (optional):** Calculated as TC minus HDL-C, this includes all "bad" cholesterol types, such as LDL-C and VLDL cholesterol.

>> **Ratio calculations:** The ratios of cholesterol components, such as TC to HDL-C or LDL-C to HDL-C, are reported to provide additional risk assessment.

TC and HDL-C are not significantly affected by food intake, so it's usually possible to take a cholesterol screening blood test at any time of day without fasting. This is not the case for TGs, however, so if your healthcare provider wants to focus more particularly on issues of TG management as part of the lipid panel measurement, it's recommended that the blood test be done when you're fasting. This may also be important if a specialist medical professional is looking at LDL-C in greater detail because high levels of TGs can affect the accuracy of LDL-C measurement.

Blood tests are usually done using a syringe and needle in a healthcare setting with the analysis undertaken in a laboratory, but rapid testing in a doctor's office or pharmacy can also be reasonably accurate. There are now commercial home finger-prick kits available, but be sure to get medical advice and to repeat more detailed analysis with more formal testing if you have any concerns about managing your cholesterol.

TIP

Get the best professional advice you can, and do the type and frequency of testing that are appropriate for you. Testing techniques provide different degrees of accuracy, and there may be some variability in results even from the same laboratory. Always remember to discuss and ask questions of your trusted, certified, and regulated healthcare provider.

Discuss the frequency and type of testing with your healthcare provider. These factors will depend on the reasons for assessing your cholesterol in the first place, your medical history, the lipid panel results, and the aims of any management strategies or treatment you may be receiving.

TIP

When you get your cholesterol or full lipid panel test, it's always a good idea to understand what's being tested and whether the result will give you and your healthcare provider the information needed to make the best assessment of the significance of the result.

Interpreting the results

If you've had a full lipid panel test at a healthcare clinic, you should be given an appointment to discuss the results with someone qualified to provide advice on the implications. You'll feel much more empowered if you're able to understand the numbers and come to a shared decision on the best management plan.

The lipid panel will provide a number of readings. The most important of these for most people is the *cholesterol ratio* (a calculation based on the levels of "good" and "bad" cholesterol). We consider this subject in more detail later in the "Paying attention to your cholesterol ratio" section, later in this chapter.

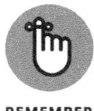

REMEMBER

High lipid levels, including high levels of LDL-C and low levels of HDL-C, are risk factors for cardiovascular disease. As such, there is no absolute cutoff for what's "normal" or "abnormal." Results always need to be considered in the context of other risk factors and the degree to which lifestyle factors may mitigate the effects of a high "bad" cholesterol level. Age also needs to be taken into account. The significance of a high cholesterol level as a risk factor for cardiovascular disease may be reasonably viewed very differently in someone in their 40s than an individual in their 80s. (We explore this subject in more detail in Chapters 7 and 8.) For someone with existing cardiovascular disease or at a particularly high risk of developing vascular disease, there are much more stringent targets for cholesterol reduction (see Chapter 11), which for the vast majority of people are achieved through medication.

Several reliable authorities advise on how to interpret a lipid panel test, including the American Heart Association (AHA), the World Health Organization (WHO), and the National Cholesterol Education Program (NCEP). The European Society of Cardiology (ESC), in collaboration with the European Atherosclerosis Society (EAS), produces guidelines about normal lipid levels and cardiovascular risk management widely used in European countries. There can be small variations in the definitions of low, optimal, or high levels of lipids between different organizations.

The usual units of measurement in the United States (milligrams/deciliter, or mg/dL) are different from those used in Europe and many other parts of the world where the results are expressed as millimoles per liter, or mmol/L.

Table 2-1 lists commonly used guidelines for lipid panel results for an average adult without a diagnosis of cardiovascular disease.

TABLE 2-1 **Cholesterol Levels Categorized**

Total Cholesterol		
Category	**mg/dL**	**mmol/L**
Optimal	Less than 200	Less than 5.2
Borderline high	200 to 239	5.2 to 6.2
High	240 or higher	≥ 6.3
LDL Cholesterol		
Category	**mg/dL**	**mmol/L**
Optimal	Less than 100	Less than 2.6
Near optimal	100–129	2.6–3.3
Borderline high	130–159	3.4–4.0
High	160–189	4.1–4.9
Very high	190 or higher	5.0 or higher

(continued)

TABLE 2-1 *(continued)*

HDL Cholesterol		
Category	**mg/dl**	**mmol/L**
Undesirably low (a risk factor)	Less than 40 for men, less than 50 for women	Less than 1.0 for men, less than 1.3 for women
High (protective)	60 or higher	1.6 or higher

Triglycerides		
Category	**mg/dL**	**mmol/L**
Normal	Less than150	Less than 1.7
Borderline high	150–199	1.7–2.2
High	200–499	2.3–5.6
Very high	500 or higher	5.7 or higher

Non-HDL Cholesterol (Total Cholesterol – HDL)		
Category	**mg/dL**	**mmol/L**
Optimal	Less than 130	Less than 3.4
Borderline High	130–159	3.4–4.0
High	160–189	4.1–4.9
Very High	190 or higher	≥ 4.9

It's important to remember that in some situations, there can be temporary changes to some of the components of a lipid panel test. If any of these situations apply, they may be reflected in the result, which is a good reason for tests to be repeated over time to make sure you have an accurate picture of your cholesterol levels in the long term.

TECHNICAL STUFF

The reasons for variability in lipid levels are quite logical. Following exercise, fats have been mobilized and consumed for energy. A temporary increase in TGs from the gut can be seen following a meal. A heart attack or other acute illness (for example, severe infection or surgery) typically causes a temporary reduction in total cholesterol, LDL, and HDL levels in what is known as the *acute phase response*, which occurs because the liver shifts focus to producing proteins that are involved in inflammation and tissue repair, instead of cholesterol. Lipid levels can remain artificially low for six to eight weeks post-illness, so retesting is recommended after recovery. Table 2-2 summarizes how various factors can affect the different lipid types.

TABLE 2-2   **Summary of Variability Effects by Lipid Type**

Factor	Total Cholesterol	LDL	HDL	Triglycerides
Recent meals	Minimal	Minimal	Minimal	Increased
Recent exercise	Minimal	Minimal	Increased	Decreased
Alcohol	Minimal	Minimal	Increased	Increased
Heart attack	Decreased	Decreased	Decreased	Decreased

WARNING

Some types of medication that you may be taking on a temporary or permanent basis can increase or decrease cholesterol levels. Your healthcare provider should be aware of any drugs you're taking.

In Chapter 4, we explore medical conditions that may alter cholesterol levels. Some of these illnesses may be temporary; after they're treated, your cholesterol levels may revert to what they were before the condition arose.

Paying attention to your cholesterol ratio

The TC/HDL ratio is a calculation that divides your TC by your HDL-C. This ratio is a marker used to assess cardiovascular risk, and it's more accurate than looking at TC alone. A high TC may not be a problem if you have a lot of beneficial HDL-C; conversely, a low TC may give false reassurance if it's composed mainly of LDL-C with very low levels of HDL-C.

A lower ratio is better because it indicates higher levels of protective HDL-C relative to TC, thereby reducing cardiovascular risk.

REMEMBER

Lipid panels are measured in mg/dL or mmol/L, but after it's converted to a ratio, the figure has no units and is universal.

Table 2-3 provides some example calculations for TC/HDL ratio using mg/dL unit measurements used in the United States. Low risk is considered anything less than 3.5, moderate risk is 3.5 to 5.0, and high risk is anything above 5.0

TABLE 2-3   **Example TC/HDL Ratios**

Risk Level	TC (mg/dL)	HDL-C (mg/dL)	Ratio (TC ÷ HDL-C)
Low	180	70	2.57
Moderate	200	50	4.0
High	250	40	6.25

BEYOND CHOLESTEROL: TAMING TRIGLYCERIDES

Triglycerides are the body's main form of stored energy, derived from the fats, carbohydrates, and proteins in food. After you eat, excess calories are converted into triglycerides and stored in fat cells for later use. Although triglycerides are vital for energy metabolism, elevated levels can contribute to cardiovascular disease and other health problems.

Triglycerides are packaged with cholesterol and proteins into *chylomicrons,* a type of lipoprotein described earlier in this chapter. Chylomicrons make their way into the bloodstream and deliver triglycerides to cells throughout the body for immediate energy use or storage. Any excess triglycerides not immediately used are taken up by the liver and either stored temporarily or repackaged into another type of lipoprotein called VLDLs. VLDLs carry triglycerides from the liver to tissues including muscle or fat cells for energy use or storage depending on what is needed in terms of energy balance.

High triglyceride levels can be an indication of excessive calorie intake, poor diet (high in sugars and refined carbohydrates), obesity, or excessive alcohol consumption. Extremely high triglyceride levels (500 mg/dL or higher, or 5.7 mmol/L or higher) also increase the risk of *acute pancreatitis,* a serious medical condition involving inflammation and potential damage to the pancreas, the organ responsible for producing insulin and digestive juices.

Although LDL cholesterol is usually the main target in lipid management, raised triglycerides have been identified as an independent risk factor for cardiovascular disease, especially in women and people with diabetes. Elevated triglycerides are a key factor for diagnosing a condition known as *metabolic syndrome,* which is a cluster of features including abdominal obesity, high blood pressure, and insulin resistance (which may include type 2 diabetes), all of which raise the risk of cardiovascular disease. (For more information on insulin resistance and type 2 diabetes, check out our other books, including *Diabetes For Dummies,* published by John Wiley & Sons.)

Beyond the Basics: Looking at Additional Tests

Most cholesterol testing and management are done by primary care providers. If you have a more complex case or higher risk, you may need to see a cardiologist to manage your cholesterol.

More advanced measurement techniques are becoming available, particularly in specialist clinics, and they may be more widely used and more comprehensively covered by health insurance in the future. Here are some tests you may be given, depending on your situation:

>> **Direct LDL-C:** This test provides a more accurate LDL-C reading, leading to more precise risk assessment and treatment decisions. It's sometimes used when triglyceride levels are very high. You don't have to fast before this test.

>> **NMR LipoProfile:** This test uses a different laboratory method to measure different types of LDL, HDL, and VLDL particles. It can, for example, identify people with high numbers of small, dense LDL particles, which are strongly associated with increased heart disease risk. (*NMR* stands for *nuclear magnetic resonance.*)

>> **Apolipoprotein B (ApoB):** This test calculates the number of lipoprotein particles that contribute most to plaque buildup in arteries. Each particle of harmful lipoprotein, including LDL and VLDL, has the common feature of containing one measurable molecule called ApoB in its structure. Counting these molecules provides a more accurate assessment of risk of cardiovascular disease compared to traditional LDL-C. This test can be particularly useful in patients with diabetes or metabolic syndrome.

Chapter **3**

Understanding High Cholesterol

I f you've ever had your cholesterol measured, you may have wondered why your cholesterol was high, average, or even perhaps reassuringly low. Your health-care provider may have discussed the factors that could be contributing to your "bad" LDL cholesterol (LDL-C) or your "good" HDL cholesterol (HDL-C). Maybe your results have changed over time, perhaps as you've made lifestyle changes or aged.

In this chapter, we explain the factors that can influence your cholesterol levels. Some are easy to modify, and others you can't do anything about. The good news is that even if reducing your cholesterol level is a challenge, you have plenty of opportunities to reduce your chances of developing cardiovascular disease.

TECHNICAL STUFF

The role of oxidation and inflammation continues to be explored by researchers because it's now understood to be a key link in the level of cholesterol and risk of developing cardiovascular disease. We cover this subject in greater detail through-out this book.

Familial High Cholesterol: Blame It on Genetics

The way you handle and metabolize fats is affected by your genetic blueprint. Genes play a significant role in regulating the production, uptake, and clearance of cholesterol in the body. High cholesterol can result from inheriting mutations in one or more genes from one or both parents.

Most people who have a high cholesterol have a multitude of dietary and environmental factors contributing to their cholesterol level. If there is a genetic predisposition as well, it's not usually a direct consequence of a single inherited gene, but more likely to be due to the combination of lifestyle factors and multiple genetic influences. This risk is called *polygenic*, and it tends to result in a moderate increase in cholesterol.

TIP

If you have a strong family history of high cholesterol levels or direct relatives have developed heart disease, stroke, or other cardiovascular diseases at an early age, perhaps without other obvious risk factors, it's definitely worth having your cholesterol checked. It may even be appropriate to have testing to see if you have a specific genetic mutation.

Here are some of the categories of high cholesterol that have a strong genetic basis:

>> **Polygenic hypercholesterolemia:** This condition results from the cumulative effect of multiple genetic variations and is not a single condition. LDL-C levels can be moderately elevated, with many small genetic contributions rather than a single dominant mutation. It may not be specifically diagnosed by genetic testing but may be inferred from a strong family history of high LDL-C or early-onset cardiovascular disease.

>> **Familial combined hyperlipidemia (FCHL):** This is a relatively common inherited disorder leading to high levels of LDL-C, VLDL-C, triglycerides, or all three. It affects about 1 percent to 2 percent of the population but is present in up to 20 percent of people with premature coronary artery disease. FCHL is likely to be the result of changes in multiple genes, with one specific named variation in a gene called USF1 being particularly common.

>> **Familial hypercholesterolemia (FH):** FH is the most well-known genetic condition linked to high cholesterol. It leads to elevated levels of LDL-C and occurs in approximately 1 in 200 to 250 people worldwide.

With FH, there are specific mutations in the LDLR gene, which encodes the LDL receptor responsible for clearing LDL-C from the blood or, less commonly, mutations in the APOB gene (affecting the ApoB protein; see Chapter 2) or the

PCSK9 gene, which normally helps regulate cholesterol levels by controlling receptors on liver cells that remove cholesterol from the blood.

The inheritance of FH is *autosomal dominant,* which means that a single copy of a mutated gene from one parent is enough to cause the condition. In heterozygous FH (which is most common), one faulty gene is inherited, and LDL levels are two to three times higher than normal. In homozygous FH, two faulty genes are inherited, one from each parent, and LDL-C levels can be four to six times higher, leading to early cardiovascular disease.

>> **Sitosterolemia:** This is a rare genetic disorder that impairs the body's ability to effectively remove plant cholesterol-like compounds called *sterols* from the bloodstream. This leads to a buildup of those sterols, which can interfere with the body's ability to regulate blood cholesterol, ultimately contributing to high levels of circulating cholesterol.

TIP

Although high cholesterol itself is usually *asymptomatic* (meaning there are no obvious visible identifiable features), there are some exceptions to this rule, especially in genetic conditions resulting in exceptionally high levels:

>> **Xanthelasma:** A condition in which yellowy, fatty deposits can be seen under the skin around the eyelids.

>> **Tendinous xanthomas:** Similar bumps or nodules around tendons, often near the elbows, knees, or Achilles tendon.

>> **Arcus corneae:** A grayish-white ring or arc that can appear around the edge of the *cornea* (the clear front part of the eye). This condition is more common in older adults in general and isn't always a sign of high cholesterol.

TIP

If you have a strong family history of high cholesterol, any of these symptoms of high cholesterol, or early onset cardiovascular disease, have your cholesterol checked early in life to rule out a genetic condition. If your levels are high, you may benefit from having further specialist investigations, including genetic testing where appropriate. The management of these conditions requires much more active treatment and almost always requires medications, as well as lifestyle modifications to reduce the risk of cardiovascular disease.

Other Causes of High Cholesterol

Long-term cholesterol increases are typically due to sustained lifestyle choices, chronic medical conditions, genetic factors, and certain medications. In this section, we cover the most common contributing factors that can lead to long-term high cholesterol and an increased risk of developing cardiovascular disease.

Diet

A diet high in saturated fats and trans fats has been linked to elevated LDL-C levels. *Saturated fats* are a type of fat that are solid at room temperature. They're present in many foods, including meat and dairy products. Trans fats are unsaturated fats that have been artificially modified through an industrial process called *hydrogenation.* This process makes fat more solid at room temperature and increases its shelf life.

TIP

Unsaturated fats (fats that are not solid at room temperature) can actually *lower* harmful LDL-C or raise beneficial HDL-C.

Other aspects of diet that adversely affect cholesterol include consuming a lot of foods that contain cholesterol (such as eggs and full-fat dairy products) and simple carbohydrates (for example, sugar, candy, and soda), as well as *ultra-processed foods* (UPFs), which are industrially manufactured products made from refined ingredients, additives, and preservatives, with minimal or no whole-food content, designed for convenience, palatability, and long shelf life. UPFs have been part of most western diets for decades and are now implicated in increasing cholesterol levels.

Lack of physical activity

A *sedentary lifestyle,* characterized by prolonged periods of inactivity, can contribute to raised LDL-C levels. Regular physical activity helps increase levels of "good" HDL-C, which plays a crucial role in removing cholesterol from the bloodstream. Inactivity can lead to lower HDL-C levels, hindering this removal process.

Sedentary behavior can also increase the triglyceride levels. Elevated triglycerides can indirectly contribute to higher LDL-C levels.

Lack of exercise can also impair the body's ability to effectively use *insulin,* the hormone responsible for regulating blood sugar. This condition, known as *insulin resistance,* can lead to metabolic changes that contribute to higher LDL-C.

Weight gain is another possible consequence of a sedentary lifestyle, which can lead to obesity and diabetes.

TIP

To manage your cholesterol, aim for at least 150 minutes per week of *aerobic exercise* (the kind of exercise that gets your heart pumping). That could be as simple as briskly walking for 30 minutes five days a week. Or combine several different types of aerobic exercise throughout the week; for example, mow the lawn with a push mower, play a game of pickup basketball, swim laps, take the stairs, hike with the dog, take a spin class, or go dancing. Exercise doesn't have to be dull!

Obesity

Weight gain, particularly when it leads to *obesity* (where too much body fat has built up to the point that it can increase the risk of health problems like heart disease, diabetes, and other chronic illnesses) can also in itself significantly impact LDL-C levels.

Excess body fat, especially *visceral fat* (fat around the organs), can trigger the liver to produce more very low-density cholesterol (VLDL-C; see Chapter 2). Obesity can interfere with the normal function of LDL receptors, which are responsible for removing LDL cholesterol from the bloodstream. When receptor activity is impaired, LDL cholesterol levels rise.

Being significantly overweight can also disrupt the body's normal metabolism of fats, which can lead to increased production of VLDL-C, which is often then converted into LDL-C. The metabolism of carbohydrates is also affected by insulin resistance resulting in increased LDL-C.

Obesity is also associated with chronic low-grade inflammation throughout the body. This inflammation can further contribute to increased LDL production and reduced LDL receptor activity, along with exacerbating the inflammation of cholesterol plaques and vascular damage.

Type 2 diabetes

Type 2 diabetes significantly impacts cholesterol levels, often leading to a condition called *diabetic dyslipidemia.* People with type 2 diabetes tend to have lower levels of "good" HDL-C. (HDL-C plays a crucial role in removing excess cholesterol from the bloodstream.) Diabetes is also strongly associated with elevated triglyceride levels; high triglycerides can interfere with the normal metabolism of cholesterol and contribute to higher LDL-C levels. In type 2 diabetes, LDL-C often exists in smaller, denser particles, which are more prone to oxidation, making them more likely to contribute to plaque buildup in the arteries (see Chapter 2). Insulin resistance, a hallmark of type 2 diabetes, can disrupt the liver's ability to properly regulate cholesterol production and removal.

Chronic kidney or liver disease

Diseases of the kidneys or liver can affect cholesterol levels, and these complications are more likely to occur with conditions such as diabetes, which is itself a risk factor for high cholesterol and cardiovascular disease.

If your kidneys aren't functioning properly, it can disrupt your body's ability to regulate cholesterol levels.

Kidney disease can also affect the production of hormones that regulate cholesterol metabolism, which can lead to increased production of LDL and decreased levels of HDL. Kidney disease can also often trigger chronic inflammation throughout the body. Inflammation can damage blood vessels and promote the development of fatty plaques and cardiovascular disease (see Chapter 4).

The liver plays a crucial role in cholesterol metabolism; if the liver is damaged, it can't effectively process cholesterol. The liver also helps remove cholesterol from the bloodstream; if the liver's function is compromised, this removal process becomes less efficient, leading to raised cholesterol levels. In some cases, liver damage can actually cause the liver to produce more cholesterol, which can further exacerbate the problem of high cholesterol.

Long-term alcohol use

The relationship between alcohol use and cholesterol is complex, and study results can be contradictory. Some research has shown that a moderate quantity of alcohol (up to one drink per day for women or two drinks per day for men) may slightly increase protective HDL-C. There are also specific compounds in red wine called *polyphenols,* which may reduce the oxidation of cholesterol. However other risks associated with alcohol use, including increased rates of many cancers, mean that you shouldn't drink alcohol in an attempt to manage your cholesterol.

WARNING

Excessive alcohol use, above current recommended limits, has negative effects on cholesterol, decreasing HDL, increasing triglycerides, and potentially causing liver damage.

Chronic stress and poor sleep

Several studies have shown that when people report high levels of chronic stress or sleep problems, they're more likely to be diagnosed with high cholesterol levels. There may be several reasons for this:

>> **There's an association between stress and poor diet, weight gain, and metabolic syndrome.** And diet, weight gain, and metabolic syndrome can cause high cholesterol.

>> **Chronic anxiety can increase levels of hormones like cortisol and adrenaline.** This can increase cholesterol and triglyceride levels, perhaps as a fight-or-flight response intended to make more fat energy sources immediately available.

>> Chronic stress is linked to chronic inflammation and *oxidative stress* (an imbalance between the production of *reactive oxygen species* (ROS) — unstable molecules that can damage cells — and the body's ability to neutralize them with antioxidants, leading to cellular and tissue damage). Oxidative stress increases the oxidation of LDL-C, which is a key component in blood vessel damage, plaque formation and rupture, and cardiovascular disease.

TIP

Chapters 9 and 10 delve more deeply into how to manage stress and achieve optimum, refreshing sleep.

Smoking and air pollution

Cigarette smoking and air pollution have a detrimental effect on cholesterol levels. Smoking raises LDL and lowers HDL, and researchers are beginning to link air pollution with similar results.

However, the biggest contribution to cardiovascular disease comes from the effects of inhaled toxins, which increase oxidative stress and chronic inflammation, and have consequences on cholesterol.

Medications

Several medications can influence lipid metabolism and cholesterol levels. Medications that can cause increased LDL, elevated triglycerides, or reduced HDL include some hormone treatments and oral contraceptives, as well as corticosteroids, anabolic steroids, and some immune-suppressing drugs (which are used, for example, following transplants or to suppress *autoimmune illnesses* — illnesses driven by the immune system). Betablockers, which are medications used for a number of conditions, including some heart-related illnesses can also adversely affect cholesterol levels.

TIP

Be sure to discuss these possible side effects with your doctor. You may have to continue taking the medication even if it raises your cholesterol, but then you may need intervention to counter this negative side effect.

Hormonal imbalances

Hormones are the chemical messengers regulating various systems in the body. They play a key role in lipid metabolism.

Here are some hormone conditions that may affect cholesterol:

» **Cushing's disease:** This condition occurs when the body produces too much of the "stress response" hormone called *cortisol.* This can increase LDL-C and decrease HDL-C.

» **Polycystic ovary syndrome (PCOS):** This condition occurs in younger women and is characterized by irregular periods, multiple small cysts in the ovaries, infertility, and sex hormone imbalance. It can increase LDL-C and decrease HDL-C.

» **Acromegaly:** This excess of growth hormone is a rare condition that's also associated with raised LDL-C and an increased risk of cardiovascular disease.

» **Thyroid disorders:** Disorders of the thyroid gland can result in reduced or increased production of the hormone thyroxine, which regulates many aspects of metabolism, heart and digestive function, muscle control, brain development, and bone health. This can lead to *hypothyroidism*, where LDL-C and triglycerides often increase, or *hyperthyroidism,* where both LDL-C and HDL-C can be reduced.

TIP

If you have a hormone condition, it's important to consider possible effects on your cholesterol and discuss them with your doctor. If your doctor is treating you for a hormone condition, they should also monitor, measure, and treat your cholesterol as necessary.

Chronic inflammatory states

Chronic inflammation not only can result in an increase in LDL-C and reduction in HDL-C, but also plays an important role in the progression of the vascular diseases linked to high cholesterol through oxidation of LDL-C, plaque instability, and the formation of damaging arterial blood clots.

Long-term low-grade inflammation can be present without any specific diagnosis through poor diet and lifestyle, obesity, and metabolic syndrome; however, it's particularly severe in disease such as rheumatoid arthritis and inflammatory bowel disease (IBD).

We cover the effects of inflammation in causing high cholesterol, as well as its progression to cardiovascular disease, in Chapter 4.

Life stages: Aging, pregnancy, and menopause

Cholesterol levels can vary at different times of life. In general, as we age, there is an increase in LDL and a reduction in HDL. This is partly a direct effect of aging, with a slowing of metabolism, but it may also be linked to changes in lifestyle (for example, a reduction in exercise). The risk associated with raised cholesterol later in life is nuanced and management decisions must take into account other quality-of-life factors. (We cover this subject in more detail in Chapter 8.)

During pregnancy, cholesterol naturally rises to support fetal development, especially in the final months. Post-pregnancy cholesterol levels generally return to normal, so there's usually no risk associated with this phenomenon and no routine measurement or treatment is advised.

Menopause often brings an increase in LDL-C and a decrease in HDL-C due to declining estrogen levels, raising the risk of cardiovascular disease.

Chapter **4**

Appreciating Oxidative Stress and Inflammation

W hen scientists first proposed a link between high cholesterol levels and *atherosclerosis* (the buildup of damaging plaques in blood vessels resulting in heart disease, stroke, and other vascular diseases), the explanation was quite simple: Too much fat in the circulating blood ended up in artery walls and eventually caused the blockages and interruptions to blood supply that resulted in damage to vital organs like the heart, brain, and kidneys, as well as the eyes, the limbs, and the rest of the body.

The story isn't that simple, though. Here's why: People with very similar cholesterol levels seem to have different risks of developing chronic diseases. This observation has led to research trying to identify the other complex factors involved.

In Chapter 1, we cover some of these other elements, such as oxidation of cholesterol and inflammation of plaques. In this chapter, we consider these important influences in more detail.

TECHNICAL STUFF

You may hear the terms *atherosclerosis* and *arteriosclerosis* used interchangeably, but there is a slight technical difference. *Atherosclerosis* refers specifically to the formation of plaques within the arterial walls due to *lipid* (fat) accumulation and inflammation; it's the primary process underlying conditions like coronary artery disease and stroke. *Arteriosclerosis* is a broader term that describes any hardening and loss of elasticity of the arteries, which can occur due to various causes, including aging or other conditions unrelated to atherosclerosis.

Looking at the Lipid Theory of Cholesterol and Chronic Disease

The association between high circulating fats (including cholesterol) and cardiovascular diseases (CVDs), and the proposed processes and steps along the way, are known as the *lipid theory* of cholesterol.

The lipid theory dates back to the mid-20th century when scientists began investigating the relationship between diet, cholesterol levels, and heart disease. One of the key figures in this research was Ancel Keys, who conducted the famous Seven Countries Study in the 1950s. His work suggested that diets high in saturated fats were associated with increased cholesterol levels and higher rates of heart disease.

Numerous other studies have confirmed this link, including the Framingham Heart Study, a long-term study showing a strong correlation between high low-density lipoprotein (LDL) cholesterol levels and the risk of heart attack and stroke.

Many scientists have challenged the methods used in some of the research that led to the lipid theory, but this criticism probably reflects the more complicated nature of the interactions and our more nuanced current understanding — it doesn't undermine the theory in its entirety. (We look at whether saturated fat can be portrayed as the villain of the story in Chapter 5.)

As more research has revealed more about the lipid theory, it has evolved over time. As long as they remain up to date, scientists and doctors are able to change their thinking and even their approach to the management of high cholesterol.

REMEMBER

Health professionals receive training in CVDs and their causes, and there is a lot of focus on cholesterol and its medical management, especially with drugs. In our experience, few doctors understand the importance of oxidation and inflammation of LDL cholesterol. It's easier to treat what we can directly measure, and oxidized LDL cholesterol isn't typically measured, so its importance is often mistakenly overlooked.

Understanding the lipid theory

In infants and children, blood vessels are elastic and flexible, with a smooth, healthy *endothelium* (the inner lining of blood vessels that efficiently regulates blood flow). The vessel walls contain minimal buildup of lipids, which eventually form plaques. In early adulthood in most people, we can detect the early stages of blood vessel wall damage from circulating lipids, and LDL deposits may be seen. Fatty streaks, the initial stage of plaque formation, can start appearing in the arterial walls, and although the blood vessels remain robust, early signs of atherosclerosis may begin in some people due to factors like diet, genetics, or lifestyle. With advancing age, plaque formation can accelerate and blood vessel walls begin to thicken with a reduction in *elastin* (the protein responsible for elasticity). This makes the vessels stiffer, which increases blood pressure. With more plaque inflammation, arteries narrow even more, resulting in decreased blood flow and the risk of clots completely blocking blood vessels, cutting off the vital supply of oxygen and nutrients to organs — a situation called *ischemia.*

You may have heard the term *ischemic heart disease,* which is the medical term for atherosclerosis in blood vessels causing heart symptoms. A transient ischemic attack (TIA) is a temporary interruption of the blood supply to the brain.

These steps are gradual and not inevitable. To reduce the risks of developing CVDs, you need to know how circulating cholesterol that's being transported to and from cells progresses to atherosclerosis and CVD. In the following sections, we provide a summary.

Excess LDL cholesterol in the bloodstream

When there is an excess of LDL cholesterol in the bloodstream, it can penetrate the endothelium. The endothelium acts as a barrier, but factors like high blood pressure, smoking, or damaging chemical reactions can damage the surface, making it possible for LDL cholesterol molecules to breach the blood vessel lining.

LDL oxidation

After LDL particles enter the *subendothelial space* (the layer of the blood vessel walls behind the protective endothelium), they're exposed to free radicals and other reactive molecules, leading to a chemical process called *oxidation.* Oxidized LDL (sometimes known as Ox-LDL) is more chemically reactive and triggers a series of harmful processes.

The damaging chemical reactions of oxidation of cholesterol starts with the presence of too many *free radicals* (highly reactive atoms or molecules with an unpaired electron) frequently in the form of a *reactive oxygen species* (ROS; free radicals whose unpaired electrons are in oxygen atoms). Oxygen's reactivity enables it to play a pivotal role in the controlled release of energy from glucose, making it an indispensable molecule for life, but in its free radical form, there's a risk of uncontrolled and damaging interactions. These free radicals contain unstable atoms with an unpaired electron, making them highly reactive and capable of damaging cells, proteins, and deoxyribonucleic acid (DNA; the molecule carrying genetic instructions for an organism's development and function) through oxidation. These oxidative processes, where free radicals "steal" electrons from other molecules to regain stable electron pairs can initiate chain reactions, where one free radical triggers the formation of additional radicals, amplifying cellular and molecular damage. The way in which antioxidants can neutralize and *reduce* free radicals is illustrated in Figure 4-1.

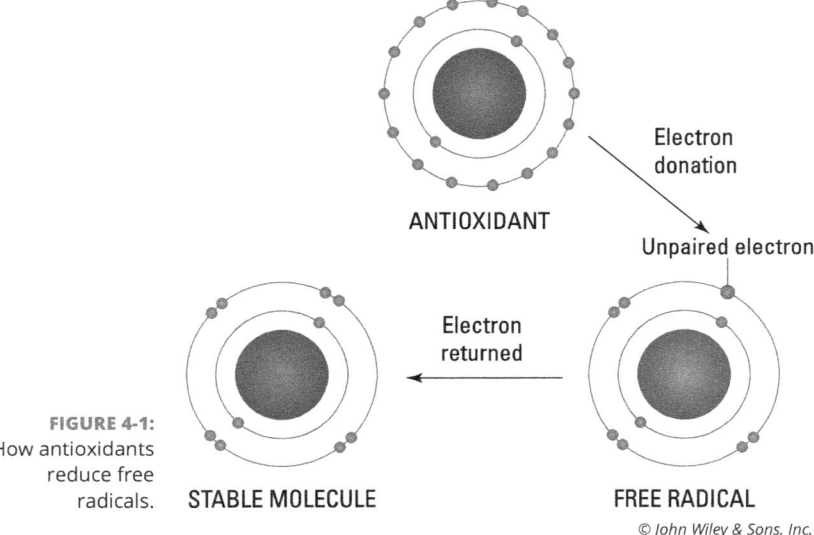

FIGURE 4-1: How antioxidants reduce free radicals.

There are always highly reactive and potentially harmful free radicals around in our bodies. They're an inevitable by-product of the trillions of chemical reactions that create energy and maintain life. Lifestyle and environmental factors also produce them. Free radicals can cause damage to molecules, numerous components of cells, and even DNA, which can result in chronic diseases. When there are excessive levels of oxidizing free radicals, the situation is called *oxidative stress.*

Oxidized LDL cholesterol is recognized as "abnormal" by the body, unlike native LDL cholesterol. This oxidized form is highly inflammatory and attracts immune cells to the site.

Endothelial injury and immune response

The presence of oxidized LDL causes the endothelium to produce warning signals so that circulating immune cells, such as *monocytes* (a type of white blood cell that acts to defend against foreign or damaged substances) adhere to the endothelial wall and migrate into the arterial wall, where they transform into *macrophages* (the body's cleanup crew). The macrophages try to remove the oxidized LDL because it's seen as "foreign" and potentially damaging.

Formation of foam cells

Inside the arterial wall, macrophages engulf the oxidized LDL particles through a process called *phagocytosis.* However, macrophages can't efficiently process the oxidized LDL. As they consume more and more oxidized LDL, they swell and transform into *foam cells,* so named because their appearance under a microscope resembles a foamy texture. Foam cells are the hallmark of early atherosclerotic plaques (also called fatty streaks). Although foam cells are part of the body's defense mechanism, their accumulation contributes to the progression of the disease.

Plaque formation

As foam cells die, they release their contents (including inflammatory substances) and cholesterol forms. These materials contribute to a growing core of lipid-rich debris within the arterial wall, which the body's protective systems recognize as needing to be managed. Muscle cells from the deeper layers of the artery are recruited to the site of damage. They proliferate and secrete fibrous proteins like collagen, which form a fibrous cap over the plaque to contain it, similar to scar tissue that forms after an injury. Over time, calcium deposits form within the plaque, further hardening it. This structure — comprising a lipid-rich core, inflammatory cells, and a fibrous cap — is known as a *mature atherosclerotic plaque.*

Plaque instability and rupture

Stable plaques, which build up over time, cause narrowing of the arteries and can restrict blood supply to vital organs. Plaque instability, on the other hand, is a critical factor in the progression to acute and sudden cardiovascular events such as heart attacks and strokes.

Heart attacks and strokes can happen when inflammatory cells within the plaque release chemicals that degrade the fibrous cap, making it thinner and more prone to rupture. As foam cells and other cells die (in a process called *necrosis*), the core of the plaque also becomes full of dead cells (called *necrotic cells*), increasing the risk of rupture.

When a plaque ruptures, its contents spill into the bloodstream. This triggers the *coagulation cascade,* leading to the formation of a blood clot (known in medical terminology as a *thrombus*). A thrombus can cause a sudden and potentially catastrophic blockage to a major artery, such as one supplying the heart or brain.

The progression of atherosclerotic plaques is illustrated in Figure 4-2.

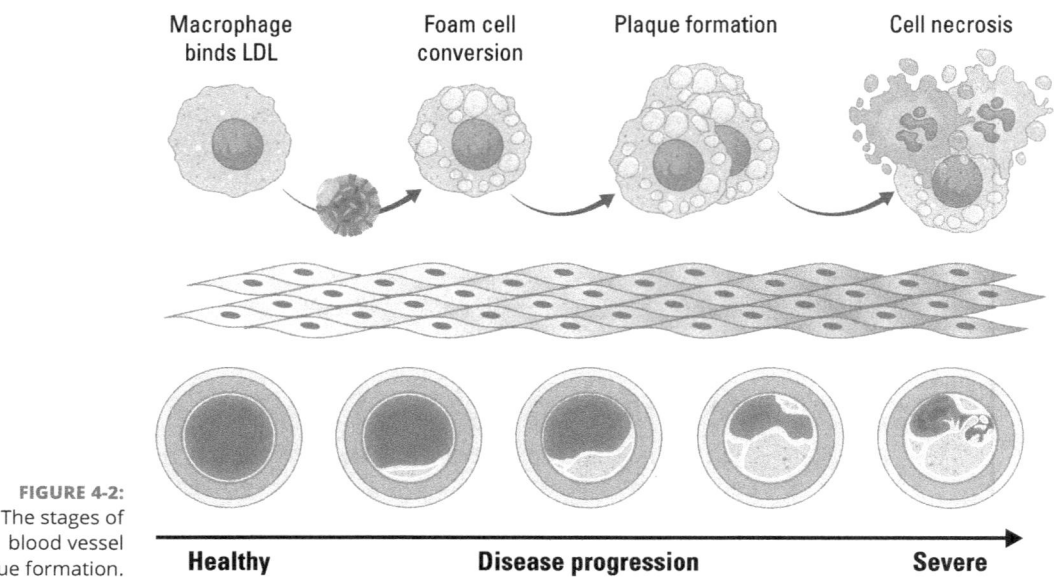

FIGURE 4-2:
The stages of blood vessel plaque formation.

REMEMBER

LDL cholesterol is not inherently harmful, but when it becomes oxidized and accumulates in the arterial wall, it triggers a vicious cycle of inflammation and plaque buildup. Foam cells, smooth muscle cells, and inflammatory signals contribute to plaque formation. Plaque instability, often driven by chronic inflammation and a thin fibrous cap, can result in life-threatening events, such as a sudden heart attack or stroke. High levels of LDL make it more likely that there will be high levels of oxidized LDL, assuming certain factors are present (for example, negative environmental and lifestyle influences) that promote oxidation and inflammation.

TIP

The successful management of cholesterol to prevent CVD should be focused on three distinct areas: cholesterol levels, the degree of cholesterol oxidation, and the drivers of inflammation. You need to consider these areas in the context of other risk factors for CVD. Many doctors and their patients concentrate solely on cholesterol, which is easily measured and easily reduced by drugs. But this approach is a huge missed opportunity for other factors to be taken into account and addressed — after all, you can have high cholesterol but low levels of oxidation and inflammation, or vice versa, which impacts your chances of developing diseased arteries.

Understanding how cholesterol leads to chronic disease

When blood vessels are damaged or narrowed by atherosclerotic plaques there's a danger that essential oxygen, glucose, and other nutrients may not get through to cells in organs performing essential tasks for life. There are three common ways in which cholesterol plaques progressing through the steps outlined in the previous section can affect blood supply:

>> **Atherosclerosis:** The gradual narrowing and loss of elasticity of blood vessels from cholesterol plaques can affect the larger blood vessels such as arteries of the *macrovascular system,* which transports blood considerable distances in the body, and the smaller arteries, called *capillaries,* which are the final vessels that interface with cells in the *microvascular system.*

>> **Aneurysm:** An *aneurysm* is a localized, abnormal bulge or ballooning in the wall of a damaged blood vessel, typically an artery, caused by a weakening of the vessel wall. If the aneurysm grows too large or ruptures, it can lead to life-threatening internal bleeding or other complications. Some aneurysms are formed as a direct result of atherosclerotic plaques.

>> **Plaque rupture:** Plaque rupture can occur if the plaque is instable. A plaque rupture usually results in a clot, which can block a major artery supplying an organ and is the most common cause of heart attacks and strokes.

If there is a slow reduction in blood supply to an organ with atherosclerosis alone, this may often be silent and insidious. It may only be picked up at a late stage when symptoms present themselves from an affected organ in distress. (We explore this subject in relation to individual diseases in the sections on the heart, brain, and other vascular diseases later in this chapter.) Plaque formation tends to occur in many arteries supplying different parts of the body, so people commonly develop multiple diseases involving several different organs.

If a plaque ruptures or an aneurysm bursts, there is more often an acute, dramatic event, which requires immediate medical support and intervention to prevent catastrophic cell death and life-threatening acute organ failure. This situation most often occurs in the form of a heart attack or stroke or a ruptured aneurysm of the main arteries running through the central abdomen, chest, or brain.

In some circumstances, there can be limited natural repair to blood vessels damaged by atherosclerosis, or following an acute rupture, the vulnerable area may be contained. If the body recognizes a gradual loss of blood supply, it's possible for new arteries to be formed above a narrowing. This process involves the growth of *collateral vessels,* which are smaller, alternative pathways that form to bypass the obstruction and restore blood flow to the affected tissue.

Measuring the effects of cholesterol

The end result of atherosclerosis can be symptoms of ischemia, which may present as pain (for example, if the heart or blood supply to a limb blood is affected) or a disturbance of consciousness (if blood vessels to the brain are impacted). It may not cause symptoms at all, especially in the early stages. Most people as they age develop varying degrees of atherosclerosis.

The extent of atherosclerosis and the effect on organ function can be measured in different ways:

» **Ultrasound:** Ultrasound is often used to visualize atherosclerotic blockages or aneurysms in larger arteries. When the technique looks at real-time changes in blood flow, it's called *Doppler ultrasound.* In a more invasive technique, ultrasound probes can be inserted into the artery to measure the size, composition, and stability of plaques even more accurately.

» **Computed tomography (CT) and magnetic resonance imaging (MRI) scans:** CTs and MRIs can also produce images of atherosclerosis and detect areas of reduced blood flow. A specialized CT scan measures calcified plaque in *coronary arteries* (the arteries supplying the heart). The amount of calcium laid down in the plaques correlates with the risk of coronary artery disease and the scan can compute a *coronary artery calcium* (CAC) *score,* which can help a doctor and patient decide how much intervention and treatment are appropriate.

» **Angiography:** Angiography involves injecting a substance into blood vessels, which are visible on X-ray, CT, or MRI scans, depending on the imaging system used. By visualizing the *contrast* (dye) picked up on the X-ray or scan, it's possible to see areas of narrowing or aneurysms. Angiography is often used to guide a physician or surgeon during interventions using techniques to locate and remove or stabilize plaques.

>> **Pulse wave velocity (PWV):** PWV measurement uses a technique involving pressure or flow sensors to assess arterial stiffness, which correlates with cardiovascular health. The more the stiffness affects flow, the greater the extent of atherosclerosis.

>> **Blood tests, electrocardiograms (EKGs), and other tests of how organs are functioning:** These tests can be used to assess the extent to which the organs may be affected by atherosclerosis, which is the end result of risk factors including high cholesterol.

Focusing on Oxidation and Inflammation

Cholesterol and other lipids have important functions, and our bodies have systems in place to transport and metabolize these molecules. In itself, circulating cholesterol is not a harmful substance. But there are factors that change an otherwise beneficial and protective component of cells into one that can build up in artery walls and threaten health.

Earlier in this chapter, we describe the importance of oxidation and inflammation in the formation and development of plaques. In general, when measured at a population level, the more circulating LDL cholesterol, the more risk there is of that cholesterol accumulating in blood vessel walls and being at risk of oxidation and inflammation, which is why there is a link between high LDL cholesterol and CVD.

However, this assumes that we all have the same level of oxidation and inflammation going on. For the same level of cholesterol measured in a standard lipid profile, two people with different lifestyles and levels of oxidative stress have very different risks of CVD. You can effectively "buck the risk" of high cholesterol. For any given level of cholesterol, the outcome for an individual can vary enormously. The trouble is, doctors use statistical, population-based models to calculate risk, and they don't measure markers of oxidation and inflammation. We explain the reasons for this situation in this section, and we explore the consequences of knowing only part of the picture when risks are assessed for management decision in Chapter 8.

Parts 2 and 4 of this book include your definitive guide to not only reducing your cholesterol ratio but also decreasing oxidation of cholesterol, oxidative stress, and inflammation, and addressing other factors that contribute to cardiovascular disease.

Oxidized cholesterol

Cholesterol can be damaged by oxidation while it's circulating or after it has built up in the subendothelial layer of blood vessels walls.

When LDL is circulating and on the move, free radical oxidation interactions with ROS (see "LDL oxidation," earlier in this chapter) tends to occur to a more limited extent, with a percentage of LDL being partially oxidized LDL.

When LDL cholesterol has been deposited and trapped in the subendothelial space, it's much more likely to be oxidized by free radicals, which are present in greater amounts. The area is very metabolically active — numerous chemical reactions take place in the cells of blood vessel walls, as well as being subject to mechanical stresses of blood flow, especially where vessels divide or branch. Oxidized LDL in the subendothelial space creates an immune response and inflammation.

Because high-density lipoprotein (HDL) collects excess cholesterol from cells, including those in artery walls, and returns it to the liver for excretion or recycling, it's less likely to become oxidized for several reasons:

>> HDL contains antioxidant enzymes that neutralize free radicals and prevent oxidative damage.

>> HDL has protective proteins that stabilize the particle and shield it from oxidative stress.

>> HDL has a higher proportion of protein relative to lipids compared to LDL, making it structurally more stable and less likely to interact with reactive species.

>> HDL's compact structure makes it less likely to get trapped in the arterial walls.

>> HDL also has anti-inflammatory effects, reducing the immune response and inflammation in blood vessels.

>> HDL encourages endothelial repair and improves the function of the arterial lining, reducing the chances of LDL penetration and retention.

HDL functionality (the ability of HDL to remove cholesterol, resist oxidation, reduce inflammation, and promote blood vessel healing and health) can vary from one person to the next. You can improve your HDL functionality with diet, exercise, and other aspects of lifestyle.

TIP

It's possible to measure circulating and endothelial oxidized LDL, as well as markers of HDL quality, but it isn't easily done, so lipid panels generally leave out this crucial indicator of what's happening to LDL and HDL. Oxidized LDL is a better indicator of atherosclerosis activity and plaque vulnerability, which are critical drivers of potentially life-threatening cardiovascular events. Circulating oxidized LDL is a marker of general oxidative stress, while endothelial oxidized LDL is an even more accurate measurement of what's happening within the blood vessel itself.

Measuring circulating or subendothelial oxidized LDL is more challenging than assessing simple LDL cholesterol because it requires specialized laboratory techniques that are less standardized and more expensive compared to traditional lipid panels. Plus, oxidized LDL levels are influenced by short-term oxidative stress, making results more variable and so arguably less suited for routine clinical use.

Oxidative stress

Oxidative stress (see Figure 4-3) occurs when there is an imbalance between the production of free radicals (most commonly ROS with unpaired electrons in oxygen atoms) and the body's ability to neutralize them with antioxidants. This imbalance leads to potential damage to lipids — especially fats in protective cell membranes, proteins, and DNA — which can damage cell structures and disrupt cellular functions, contributing to various diseases. LDL cholesterol is particularly susceptible to oxidation in situations of oxidative stress, resulting in atherosclerosis. Lipids in cell membranes of the brain are also especially vulnerable.

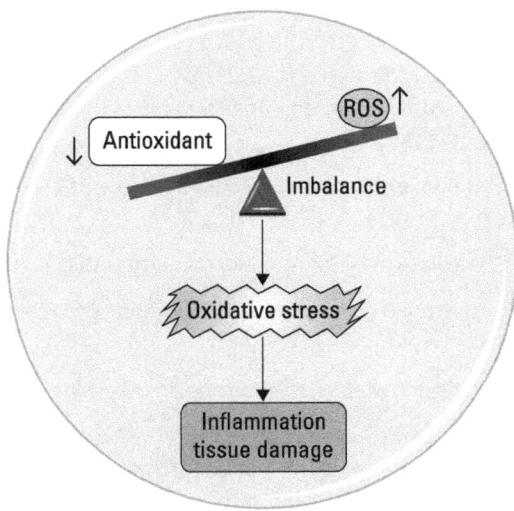

FIGURE 4-3:
Oxidative stress in a cell.

© John Wiley & Sons, Inc.

A good way to picture the potential reactivity of free radicals is to consider one of the most common forms of ROS generated in the body: hydrogen peroxide. You've probably heard of the use of hydrogen peroxide in certain highly concentrated forms for chemical industrial cleaning, bleaching, metal breakdown, and even in rocket fuel. No wonder it's important for our bodies to have mechanisms in place for neutralizing free radicals like this efficiently and quickly.

Our bodies have evolved intricate systems to counteract oxidative stress and maintain a balance. This is sometimes referred to as the *redox system.* A robust antioxidant system can mitigate ROS damage effectively by reversing or counter-ing the chemistry with the opposite of oxidation — using antioxidant molecules, which are free to donate electrons to unpaired oxygen atoms in the process oppo-site to oxidation called *reduction.* Unfortunately, sometimes reduction isn't enough.

REMEMBER

When the term *oxidative stress* is used, it's generally a reference to a net imbalance, with the factors driving oxidative stress outweighing those that our bodies employ to reduce uncontrolled chemical oxidation pathways.

Your genes can affect your ability to reduce oxidative stress, and the efficiency of your redox system reduces with age. In general, however, keeping oxidative stress at bay is achieved by reducing those modifiable factors that increase it, and by supporting and boosting your body's defensive systems.

WARNING

Here are the most important factors that increase ROS and may lead to oxidative stress in the long term if they persist:

>> **Internal causes:** Free radicals are naturally produced within the body through normal processes, including energy production by cells, digestion and metabolism, and inflammation.

>> **Environmental pollution:** Exposure to pollutants like ozone, nitrogen oxides, and particulate matter increase ROS.

>> **Ultraviolet (UV) radiation:** Solar radiation generates ROS in the skin.

>> **Smoking:** Tobacco smoke contains free radicals and chemicals that stimulate their production.

>> **Alcohol consumption:** Metabolism of alcohol in the liver generates ROS.

>> **Unhealthy diet:** High intake of processed foods, trans and saturated fats, chargrilled ingredients, an excess of refined carbohydrates and simple sugars, animal protein overloaded diets, and possibly a diet high in vegetable oils introduces a higher proportion of ROS. Low-fiber diets also increase the levels of ROS.

>> **Exposure to toxins:** Pesticides, heavy metals (like mercury or lead), and industrial chemicals can trigger free radical formation.

>> **Radiation:** Ionizing radiation from medical imaging or nuclear sources directly generates ROS.

>> **Stress and sleep deprivation:** Psychological and physical stressors may increase ROS production.

TIP

Avoiding these factors that increase free radicals is important for reducing oxidative stress. Avoid excess radiation from whatever source and quit harmful substances (like unhealthy ROS-generating foods, tobacco, and excess alcohol). Use sunscreen when you're getting prolonged exposure to UV light, and wear an N99 or FFP3 mask in specifically risky environments to avoid inhaling toxic particles as well.

TIP

The body regulates free radical levels through antioxidant defense systems. Here are factors that control ROS:

>> **Internal protective redox systems:** Chemicals that act as antioxidants, break down ROS, or contribute to the repair of damaged oxidized cell membranes or internal structures all contribute directly or indirectly to reducing the damage of oxidative stress.

>> **Healthy diet:** The most important external counterbalance to oxidative stress comes from a healthy diet. Fats like oleic acid, some vitamins and minerals, and bioactive compounds including polyphenols (see Chapter 6) all can have beneficial antioxidant effects.

>> **Good-quality sleep:** Improved sleep and psychological factors can reduce oxidative stress (see Chapter 9).

>> **Exercise:** Regular exercise, despite causing temporary ROS spikes with increase metabolism, leads to stronger antioxidant defenses, reduced chronic inflammation, and overall improved net oxidative balance. Regular physical activity is a key strategy for minimizing oxidative stress and promoting long-term health.

Inflammation

The response of the immune system and the chronic inflammation that may follow is a key step in the formation of atherosclerotic plaques. Progression from a stable plaque to an unstable plaque can also be driven by inflammation.

Inflammation is actually a vital response of the body to injury or infection. In its acute form, inflammation is protective and helps the body heal. For example, when you cut your finger, the area may become red, swollen, and warm. This reaction is acute inflammation, a short-term process where immune cells, such as white blood cells, rush to the site to eliminate pathogens, clear debris, and initiate repair. Acute inflammation resolves when the healing process is complete, ensuring that tissues return to their normal state.

Chronic inflammation, on the other hand, is a harmful, long-term process. Instead of resolving, the inflammatory response persists and can cause damage to healthy tissues. This often happens when the body mistakenly triggers the immune system or fails to regulate it properly. Chronic inflammation is associated with a wide range of diseases, including diabetes, rheumatoid arthritis, and CVDs like atherosclerosis.

The contrast between acute and chronic inflammation is shown in Figure 4-4.

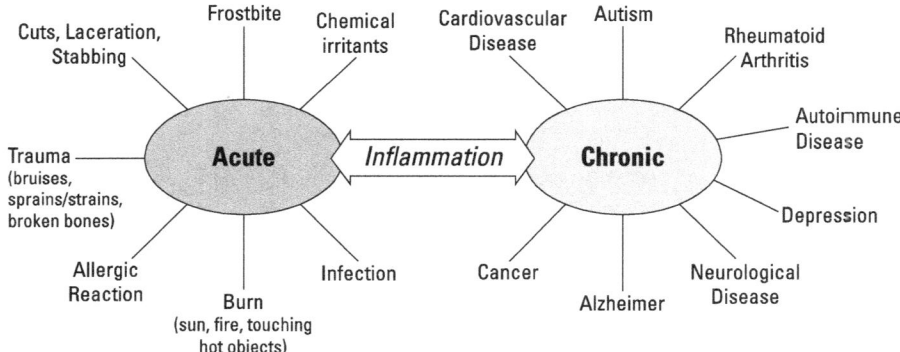

FIGURE 4-4: The difference between acute and chronic inflammation.

© John Wiley & Sons, Inc.

In the processes involved in atherosclerosis, LDL cholesterol becomes oxidized in the walls of blood vessels, and the body treats oxidized LDL as harmful, triggering an inflammatory response. Immune cells are recruited to engulf the oxidized LDL, forming foam cells, which accumulate in the arterial walls and lead to the formation of the characteristic plaques of atherosclerosis. Unlike the self-limiting nature of acute inflammation, the ongoing presence of oxidized LDL keeps the inflammatory response active, perpetuating tissue damage and promoting disease progression, arterial narrowing, and plaque instability.

The localized oxidation of LDL is also influenced by *systemic* factors — those that affect the whole body. It's made worse when there's a generalized state of oxidative stress, where the drivers of oxidation (such as smoking and poor diet) are not adequately balanced or regulated.

Similarly, there can be a systemic *proinflammatory* state, in which inflammatory signals dominate and drive a cycle of immune activation and tissue injury. Several factors promote inflammation in the body and are similar to those that cause oxidative stress. These include smoking, a diet high in refined carbohydrates, excess alcohol, obesity, chronic stress, and environmental pollutants. Conversely, anti-inflammatory factors can help restore balance and protect the body. These include a diet rich in fruits, vegetables, nuts, seeds, and fatty fish, which provide antioxidants and omega-3 fatty acids. Regular physical activity, stress management, adequate sleep, and avoiding smoking or excessive alcohol consumption also support anti-inflammatory processes.

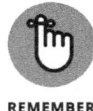

REMEMBER

Oxidative stress and chronic inflammation are distinct processes, but they're interconnected. Oxidative stress can amplify inflammation, and chronic inflammation can increase oxidative stress.

In the same way that it would be very useful to know your circulating oxidized LDL levels, having a measurement of the amount of systemic inflammation would provide an indication of the risk of progression of atherosclerosis for any level of cholesterol reported in your full lipid panel. Doctors often measure specific *inflammatory markers* in the blood like C-reactive protein (CRP) to diagnose and monitor inflammatory diseases, such as infections, autoimmune disorders, or conditions like rheumatoid arthritis. In research settings, higher-sensitivity tests are used to detect low levels of inflammation that indicate more subtle, systemic, or chronic inflammation not easily detected by conventional tests. These are particularly important for studying proinflammatory states and their role in chronic diseases like CVD, which have an inflammatory basis. Tests like high-sensitivity CRP (hs-CRP) and cytokines are not yet used widely to assess the risk of developing CVD, but they may have a role in the future.

Identifying the Diseases Caused by High Cholesterol

The effects of plaque formation in the walls of blood vessels from LDL cholesterol undergoing oxidation and inflammation include narrowing of the vessels and reduced blood supply to organs. This process occurs gradually over time, resulting in loss of oxygen and nutrient supply to the cells of the body that perform the tasks essential for life, and the consequence can be an organ failing in its functions.

Sometimes, plaques become unstable. The fibrous cap (the outer covering) can get thin and weak because of inflammation and stress from blood flow. If the cap breaks open and ruptures, the inside of the plaque, made up of fatty material and proteins, gets exposed to the blood. When this happens, the body reacts by trying to "patch" the damaged area. Platelets, the tiny cells in blood that help with clotting, stick to the exposed plaque and clump together. This triggers a chain reaction where the blood thickens and clots to seal the break. The process is called *thrombosis,* and the clot itself is a *thrombus.* Such a clot or thrombus can grow big enough to block the artery completely; this can happen very quickly, creating an acute and immediate threat to the blood supply to an organ.

In addition to forming directly at the site of a ruptured plaque, clots (or parts of them) can sometimes break loose and travel through the bloodstream. These moving clots, called *emboli,* are carried along by the blood until they reach a smaller artery that they can't pass through, causing a blockage in that localized area. This process, called *thromboembolism,* highlights how clots can cause harm even away from the original site of plaque rupture.

Heart attack

When atherosclerosis occurs in blood vessels that supply the heart, areas of heart muscle can suffer from poor blood supply. This can lead to *heart failure,* when the muscle of the heart is starved of the blood supply needed to keep it functioning effectively in pumping blood around the body. It may also present with symptoms such as *angina,* where the strain on the heart shows up with chest pain especially on exertion, when demands on the heart are greatest.

Healthy blood vessels supplying the heart are illustrated in Figure 4-5. Heart disease occurs when these blood vessels develop significant atherosclerosis.

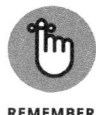

REMEMBER

Ischemia is the medical term used when there is an inadequate blood supply to a tissue or organ, resulting in reduced oxygen and nutrient delivery needed for normal function and survival. This condition may be temporary and can be reversed with medical interventions. Ischemic heart disease is the most common form of cardiovascular illness.

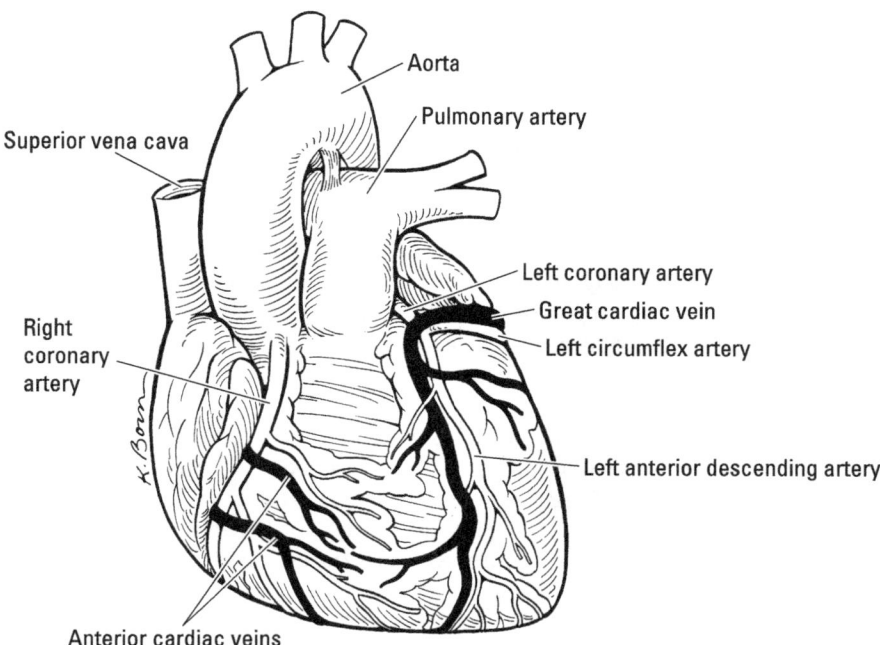

FIGURE 4-5: Blood vessels in a healthy heart.

When a thromboembolism occurs with plaque rupture, it can create a sudden blockage of one of the main arteries supplying blood to the heart. *Infarction* refers to tissue death caused by a prolonged lack of blood supply, resulting in severe and critical oxygen and nutrient deprivation. If a sudden thromboembolic event occurs, it can result in a *myocardial infarction* (heart attack), in which heart muscle dies.

Stroke

If there is a more acute blood vessel blockage with a thrombus or thromboembolic event, it usually presents with more sudden symptoms. These may be weakness or numbness, especially on one side of the body, difficulty speaking or understanding speech, vision problems, severe headache, or loss of coordination and balance. The specific symptoms depend on the area of the brain affected by the reduced blood flow.

This can be temporary and reversible, in which case it's called a *transient ischemic attack* (TIA). If the damage is permanent, it's called a *cerebrovascular accident* (CVA) or, more commonly, a stroke.

When there's a gradual reduction in adequacy of blood supply to the brain, it can affect *cognition* (a person's ability to think and process information) and result in vascular dementia.

Other vascular diseases

WARNING

Atherosclerosis can occur in any blood vessel, large or small, supplying any area of the body. It often affects many organs at the same time. Doctors investigating and treating patients with ischemic heart or cerebrovascular disease will look for evidence of other blood vessels being affected in a similar way, to prevent and treat further changes.

Gradual or sudden loss of blood supply to limbs can be the result of *peripheral vascular disease* (changes in the blood vessels supplying more distant parts of the body). This can present with pain in the legs when walking or more acutely with sudden color changes and coldness of the skin when a sudden blockage occurs. Without timely intervention, tissue death may result and the limb may develop gangrene.

The kidneys are especially dependent on good blood supply to perform the tasks of clearing waste products from circulation. Unchecked atherosclerosis and thromboembolic events in the *renal* blood vessels (those in the kidneys) can insidiously or more acutely cause long-term kidney disease or kidney failure, resulting in the buildup of toxic waste products in the body.

The eyes need a rich supply of blood, especially through the complex network of tiny blood vessels supplying the retina. An optician should check the backs of your eyes regularly and refer you to a specialist if there's evidence of atherosclerosis, which may cause problems with vision.

The blood supply to a large section of the digestive tract is through an artery called the *mesenteric artery*. If this artery becomes blocked, it can cause sudden abdominal pain and often requires lifesaving surgery to preserve parts of the gut, which may die if there's not enough blood getting through.

REMEMBER

These are just a few examples of the importance of atherosclerosis and its potential effects on different arteries and organs.

The special case of diabetes

Diabetes is especially associated with atherosclerosis because high blood glucose over time can damage the inner lining of blood vessels, making it easier for cholesterol and other harmful substances to stick to the walls. This leads to the buildup of plaques, which narrow the arteries and restrict blood flow.

High blood glucose levels in people with diabetes can interfere with the body's ability to manage cholesterol properly, increasing LDL cholesterol, lowering HDL cholesterol, and causing changes in the way HDL functions, making it less effective at removing cholesterol from the arteries. High blood glucose can also make LDL particles more likely to become oxidized, which is particularly harmful and pro-inflammatory.

People with type 2 diabetes tend to have higher levels of systemic inflammation, which can worsen the damage to blood vessels. In addition, diabetes often causes changes in the blood, such as increased clotting, which makes it more likely for blood clots to form. Combined, these factors speed up the development of atherosclerosis, increasing the risk of serious health problems like heart attacks, strokes, and other forms of vascular disease, including problems with vision and kidney disease. Keeping blood glucose levels in check is key to reducing these risks and protecting heart and brain health, as well as the other conditions associated with poorly controlled diabetes.

We've written extensively on the subject of diabetes. You can find more information in *Diabetes For Dummies, Diabetes Meal Planning & Nutrition For Dummies, Diabetes Cookbook For Dummies,* and *Diabetes Desserts Cookbook For Dummies* (all published by John Wiley & Sons, Inc.).

2

Changing Your Diet to Manage Cholesterol

IN THIS PART . . .

Identify foods that affect cholesterol.

Learn the role of cholesterol in the diet.

Discover cholesterol-friendly foods.

Choose fiber, healthy fats, and stanols.

Appreciate the role of polyphenols.

Consider the importance of a healthy gut microbiome.

Chapter **5**

Understanding the Role of Cholesterol and the Diet

C holesterol is present in a number of different foods, but most *circulating cholesterol* (the cholesterol in the blood) is made in the liver from other fats in the diet and is influenced by many other factors. Although the body regulates the amount of cholesterol manufactured and recycled or broken down, too much of certain types of dietary fats, including trans fats and some saturated fats, can result in high levels of circulating low-density lipoprotein (LDL) cholesterol.

In the past, healthcare professionals recommended that people cut down on cholesterol-containing foods, eliminate trans fats, and reduce saturated fat, but that advice has evolved in recent years. Now we know that there are different subtypes of saturated fats, some of which don't seem to raise cholesterol, and there are beneficial types of unsaturated fats that lower the cholesterol ratio by reducing LDL and increasing high-density lipoprotein (HDL) cholesterol.

Perhaps even more important, new evidence has shown that cholesterol levels are affected by almost every aspect of the diet, not just the fats we consume. For example, refined carbohydrates and some ingredients of processed foods can adversely affect regulation of circulating cholesterol. Replacing fats in the diet with carbohydrates isn't healthy if those carbs are refined and cause weight gain, promoting diabetes and inflammation, or if the low-fat option is full of chemicals that might have a harmful effect on cholesterol or its level of oxidation.

The good news is that, in addition to unsaturated fats, there are other nonfat constituents in foods that can reduce harmful LDL cholesterol and boost HDL cholesterol.

Finally, you can incorporate in your diet important foods that have powerful antioxidant and anti-inflammatory properties. We may not be able to easily measure the reduction in *oxidized* LDL, but the effect can be to significantly reduce the likely level of harm for any given level of cholesterol.

In this chapter, you begin to appreciate the connection between your diet and your cholesterol level. You also discover how to maximize protective foods that can play an important part in reducing the oxidation and inflammation of LDL cholesterol.

Identifying Foods That Raise Cholesterol

Some foods are known to raise cholesterol and increase oxidative stress (see Chapter 4), and when you know what those foods are, you can eliminate or avoid them. In this section, we walk you through the list. Think of this section as a map pointing out all the landmines to avoid along your journey.

TIP

The old adage "Everything in moderation" is often quoted when it comes to nutrition. Although the sentiment is designed to prevent excess, the phrase is misleading. Foods that are overtly unhealthy and unnecessary can and should be eradicated from our diets and replaced with much better tasting, healthy, and natural substitutes. Sodas (whether full sugar or artificially sweetened) and ultra-processed convenience foods don't need to be eaten in moderation — they shouldn't be eaten at all.

Trans fats

Trans fats were first introduced into the food supply in the early 20th century as a way to make vegetable oils solid at room temperature, which made them useful for products like margarine, baked goods (cookies, cakes, pastries), and some snack foods. Trans fats are also created in some cooking processes (see "Foods cooked at high temperatures," later in this chapter).

Initially, they were considered a *healthier* alternative to saturated fats, but research in the 1990s began to reveal the harmful effects of trans fats on heart health.

Today we known that trans fats cause a significant increase in LDL cholesterol and increase the risk of cardiovascular disease (CVD).

It's estimated that trans fats have caused tens of thousands of premature deaths from heart disease in the United States alone. In response to these findings, many countries have implemented regulations to limit or ban the use of trans fats in food products. Many European countries, Canada, and the United States led with stricter rules and have been followed by others. The World Health Organization (WHO) is actively promoting the global elimination of trans fats, and more countries are joining the effort to protect public health.

Saturated fats

Saturated fats have the potential to affect cholesterol. Many, but not all, saturated fats increase LDL cholesterol more than HDL cholesterol, though some can actually raise HDL more than LDL, which may benefit the overall cholesterol ratios (see the nearby sidebar).

Fats are used in the body as a source of energy, for building cell membranes, producing hormones, and providing insulation and protection for organs. Fats can be *saturated* or *unsaturated*; unsaturated fats include *monounsaturated* and *polyunsaturated*.

Saturated fats are solid at room temperature, like butter. Monounsaturated fats, on the other hand, are liquid at room temperature, such as olive oil. Polyunsaturated fats are very fluid, as seen in fish oil.

TIP

You can find more on unsaturated fats in the "Appreciating healthy fats and stanols" section, later in this chapter.

TECHNICAL
STUFF

DIGGING DEEP INTO CHEMISTRY

Fats most commonly exist in the form of three fat acid molecules made up of carbon (C), hydrogen (H), and oxygen (O) atoms in triglycerides, which consists of one glycerol molecule that acts as a three-carbon backbone and three fatty-acid chains. The fatty-acid chains are long chains of carbon atoms with hydrogen atoms attached, and they have a carboxyl group (-COOH) at one end that connects to the glycerol.

Saturated fats have fatty acid chains in which all the carbon atoms are "saturated" with hydrogen, meaning there are no double bonds between the carbons; this gives them a straight structure, allowing them to pack tightly together, which makes them

(continued)

(continued)

solid at room temperature. Monounsaturated fats, on the other hand, have one double bond in the carbon chain, which reduces the number of hydrogen atoms; the double bond creates a slight bend in the chain, preventing tight packing, so they're liquid at room temperature. Polyunsaturated fats have two or more double bonds in their carbon chains, resulting in even fewer hydrogen atoms; these multiple double bonds cause bends or kinks in the chains, making them very fluid.

The structure of triglycerides is consistent in having a glycerol backbone, but the properties and health effects of fats vary depending on the types of fatty acid chains attached. For example, butter mostly contains triglycerides with saturated fatty acids, while olive oil is rich in triglycerides with monounsaturated fats.

There are several different subtypes of saturated fat. The length of fatty-acid chains influences their impact on cholesterol levels. Short- and medium-chain saturated fatty acids, such as those found in coconut oil (for example, caprylic and capric acids), are quickly metabolized for energy and have minimal effects on LDL or HDL cholesterol. In contrast, long-chain saturated fatty acids (like palmitic and myristic acids) significantly raise LDL cholesterol and, although they also increase HDL cholesterol, it's to a lesser extent, so the overall cholesterol ratio is raised. Stearic acid, another long-chain fatty acid, is an exception: It has little to no effect on cholesterol levels because it's often converted into oleic acid in the body.

Generally, the longer the fatty acid chain, the greater its potential impact on increasing LDL cholesterol, with some variability based on the specific fatty acid.

TIP

If a saturated fat raises both LDL and HDL, the conclusion about whether it's a "good" or "bad" saturated depends on whether it raises "bad" LDL more than "good" HDL or vice versa. In other words, its net effect on the cholesterol ratio (see Chapter 3). Table 5-1 lists some examples of saturated fats, their most common food sources and their effects on LDL and HDL cholesterol.

TABLE 5-1   ## Saturated Fats and Their Effect on Cholesterol

Saturated Fat Type	Common Sources	Effect on LDL Cholesterol	Effect on HDL Cholesterol
Lauric acid	Coconut oil, palm kernel oil, dairy	Moderate increase	Moderate increase
Myristic acid	Butter, cheese, milk fat, coconut	Significant increase	Significant increase
Palmitic acid	Palm oil, meat, dairy products	Significant increase	Neutral effect or slight increase
Stearic acid	Dark chocolate, meat, cocoa butter	Neutral effect	Neutral effect or slight increase
Capric and caprylic acid	Coconut oil, medium-chain triglyceride (MCT) oil, goat's milk	Neutral effect or minimal increase	Neutral effect or minimal increase

Refined carbohydrates

The type and quality of carbohydrates influence cholesterol levels, which is one of the reasons why the outdated public health advice to reduce fat and increase carbohydrate consumption, without making distinctions about the type of fats and carbohydrates, was flawed. Refined, simple sugars — like high-fructose corn syrup, white or brown granulated or caster sugar, white rice, and white bread— can lower HDL cholesterol and increase triglycerides.

Excess alcohol

A modest amount of alcohol can increase HDL, with antioxidants in red wine possibly reducing the oxidation of cholesterol, but increased alcohol consumption causes a rise in LDL and triglycerides. Alcohol can have other harmful effects on health as well.

Processed foods

Foods manufactured by industrial processes to specifically appeal to consumers for their taste and convenience often have additives to improve texture and lengthen shelf life. Some estimates suggest that as much as 50 percent of calories in a typical western diet come from such *ultra-processed foods*. (See the nearby sidebar for more.)

Research into these ingredients is relatively new, but already some worrying trends have been identified. The current thinking is that artificial ingredients in processed foods can negatively impact cholesterol levels in several ways. For example, emulsifiers may disrupt the gut microbiome, leading to inflammation that may increase LDL cholesterol and impair cholesterol metabolism (see "Grasping the role of the gut microbiome," later in this chapter for more on the gut microbiome). Artificial sweeteners such as aspartame and sucralose can also alter gut bacteria, potentially lowering HDL cholesterol and contributing to *dyslipidemia* (unhealthy levels of lipids such as cholesterol and triglycerides in the blood). Synthetic antioxidants like butylated hydroxytoluene (BHT) and butylated hydroxyanisole (BHA), which are used to extend shelf life in packaged foods, may interfere with lipid metabolism and increase cholesterol imbalances.

ULTRA-PROCESSED FOODS: WHAT TO LOOK OUT FOR

Not all foods are obviously ultra-processed. A good example of this is a staple of many people's diet: bread. You can buy freshly baked bread with just four ingredients: flour, water, yeast, and a little salt. (It may also include added vitamins and minerals.) But some commercial breads have as many as 16 or more added ingredients for texture and shelf life, which can include emulsifiers, sugars, colorants, preservatives, and artificial flavors.

Some foods may appear to be ultra-processed, but when you look at the ingredient list, you may be pleasantly surprised. Some manufacturers are trying to "clean up" the food environment and use only natural ingredients (for example, using ascorbic acid, which is vitamin C, instead of nitrites as a preservative). Other examples include the use of olive oil or herbs and spices as natural preservatives and a plant wall compound called *pectin* used as a stabilizer of foods. Natural colors found in fruits and vegetables can replace artificial food dyes.

Here's a list of common ultra-processed foods:

- **Sugary drinks:** These include sodas, fruit juices (if they have added sugars or other ingredients), sports drinks, energy drinks.

- **Packaged snacks:** Examples include chips, crackers, cookies, candy, processed popcorn, premade trail mix with candy or chocolate.

- **Ready-to-eat meals:** These include frozen meals, instant noodles, premade pasta dishes, and microwaveable meals.

- **Processed meats:** These include hot dogs, sausages, bacon, deli meats (like ham and salami), jerky.

- **Breakfast cereals:** Many breakfast cereals, especially those marketed to children, are high in sugar and low in fiber.

- **Fast food:** Examples include burgers, fries, chicken nuggets, pizza (especially commercially prepared versions).

- **Baked goods:** These include cakes, cookies, pastries, donuts (especially commercially produced ones).

- **Ice cream and frozen desserts:** Many commercial ice creams and frozen desserts contain a long list of added ingredients.

- **Protein bars and shakes:** Some can be healthy, but many are high in sugar, artificial sweeteners, and other additives.

- **Imitation meats and cheeses:** These often contain numerous additives to mimic the taste and texture of real meat or cheese.

- **Sauces and dressings:** Many commercially prepared sauces and dressings are high in sugar, salt, and other additives.

Apps such as Yuka (`https://yuka.io`) provide reliable information on food additives. Just scan the product's bar code with your phone, and the app will tell you the current state of research concerning all the ingredients, summarizing the food as excellent, good, poor, or bad.

Foods that increase oxidative stress and inflammation

Refined carbohydrates — including added sugars like high-fructose corn syrup — can contribute to oxidative stress and inflammation because of their impact on blood glucose and insulin. Such foods are described as *pro-inflammatory*. Unhealthy fats, including trans fats and some saturated fats are also linked to inflammatory processes. A high ratio of omega-6 polyunsaturated fat to omega-3 polyunsaturated fat is also now known to be a driver of inflammation. Artificial sweeteners and processed meats may further promote inflammation and oxidative stress.

Foods cooked at high temperatures

Foods cooked at high temperatures can produce harmful compounds that are pro-inflammatory and increase oxidative stress.

TECHNICAL STUFF

Advanced glycation end products (AGEs), polar compounds, heterocyclic amines (HCAs), polycyclic aromatic hydrocarbons (PAHs), advanced lipoxidation end products (ALEs), and aldehydes like acrolein are examples of chemicals that can increase oxidation and inflammation of cholesterol plaques, in addition to having other systemic effects.

Foods high in protein and fat — such as red meat, skin on poultry, and fried items — tend to produce more harmful compounds like HCAs, PAHs, and AGEs when cooked at high temperatures. This is because their composition provides the necessary building blocks for these compounds, and high-heat cooking methods accelerate their formation, especially when oxidizing free radicals are generated.

Conversely, vegetables and fruits, with their lower protein and fat content, higher water content, and abundance of antioxidants, generally produce fewer of these undesirable compounds during cooking.

Although the food itself is the largest contributor to these compounds, it's also important to remember that cooking oil can contribute to or inhibit the production of these chemicals. Cooking oils and fats high in polyunsaturated fatty acids, like many vegetable oils, are more prone to breaking down and forming harmful compounds at high temperatures. Oils and fats with fewer antioxidants also offer less protection against the formation of these compounds in foods during cooking. This is why extra-virgin olive oil is the best oil for cooking (see Chapter 6).

Excess salt

In some people, excess salt in the diet can lead to increased blood pressure. Although high blood pressure doesn't have a direct impact on cholesterol levels, the result may be increased stiffness of blood vessel walls with a heightened risk of injury to the lining of the vessels, known as the *endothelium*. This disruption can be a step in the process of plaque formation because LDL cholesterol is much more likely to accumulate and undergo oxidation in a damaged part of the blood vessel wall. High levels of salt can also be proinflammatory.

TIP

READING FOOD LABELS

Get into the habit of looking at food labels to make the best decisions about what you're buying and eating. Information on foods can take many forms — advertising, approved health claims, and nutritional information. In most countries, this food labelling is regulated by standards and legal requirements.

Some of the information on labels, even official guidelines, is quite simplistic and limited. The label may list saturated fat, but the different *subtypes* of saturated fat are not usually listed. Warnings about additives and preservatives aren't typically included in nutritional guidelines. Beneficial nutritional qualities such as the presence of compounds like polyphenols are not listed. Calories are often listed, but most experts in nutrition agree that calorie counting in itself is not a very useful indication of the tendency to promote weight gain or diseases. Nutritional information can be useful as a guide, but it's also important to read the ingredient list.

The ingredient list may be daunting at first — you may need to take your reading glasses with you to the supermarket! Most countries require every ingredient to be listed on the labels of packaged foods, unless the amounts are negligible. In general, fresh fruits and vegetables don't need to be labeled, for good reason: A carrot is a carrot, and an orange is an orange!

Reading ingredients lists makes it possible to avoid or substantially reduce your intake of the foods that negatively impact cholesterol and, in the process, improve your cholesterol profile. When you get used to interpreting ingredients, you'll find it much easier to make the best choices and be empowered to gain mastery over your cholesterol.

TECHNICAL STUFF

CHOLESTEROL AND SATURATED FAT CONTROVERSIES

The lipid theory (see Chapter 4) links dietary saturated fat to CVD through increased LDL cholesterol. But in the 1980s, data seemed to suggest that, despite a diet high in saturated fat, the people of some regions of France had low death rates from heart disease. This phenomenon was called the *French paradox*. A theory to explain this apparent contradiction to the lipid theory emerged, suggesting that the benefits of moderate red wine for health counteracted the negative effects of saturated fat in the French diet. According to current thinking, what's more likely is that the supposedly lower CVD death rates were inaccurate, due to a flawed recording of the cause of death.

More recently, however, research, including the large-scale Prospective Urban Rural Epidemiology (PURE) study, published in the *Lancet* in 2017, has again challenged the long-held belief that reducing saturated fat intake improves heart and vascular health. The PURE study found that higher intakes of total and saturated fat were not significantly associated with increased CVD risk and were even linked to lower mortality, whereas high carbohydrate consumption was correlated with worse health outcomes.

Despite the provocative findings of the PURE study, which has been followed by heated debate among scientists and in the media, mainstream health authorities haven't changed their dietary recommendations, partly because the study has been criticized for its limitations, including reliance on self-reported dietary data, variations in food availability across different populations in the study, and potential confounding factors that make it difficult to prove the cause and effect suggested by the study. (*Confounding*

(continued)

(continued)

factors are other influences that can make it hard to tell if one thing, like diet, is really causing a health effect or if something else is playing a role.) Many experts argue that well-controlled trials and long-term studies still support the link between saturated fat, elevated LDL cholesterol, and increased CVD risk, reinforcing the current guidelines that emphasize reducing saturated fat intake in favor of unsaturated fats and whole foods for heart health.

These findings suggest that dietary guidelines focusing on fat reduction may be overly simplistic and that other factors, such as carbohydrate quality, overall diet composition, the complex composition of whole foods, and metabolic health, play crucial roles in cardiovascular risk. It also likely reflects the fact that not all saturated fats raise cholesterol and the oxidation of LDL. Plus, systemic drivers of oxidative stress and inflammation are not adequately measured and assessed despite their impact on the risk of CVD.

This book considers *all* the contributing factors, embraces the complexity of the debate, and provides the best advice about the foods you can enjoy and that are known to lower cholesterol, reduce oxidized LDL, and diminish the risk of CVD.

LOOKING AT WHOLE FOODS

Natural foods are more than their main macronutrients. For example, it would be misleading to describe cheese simply as a saturated fat and to conclude that it must cause a rise in cholesterol, be a risk for CVD, and be eliminated from our diets. Cheese is also a source of protein and carbohydrates. The health of full-fat dairy is a subject of debate. Although full-fat dairy is high in saturated fats, some of which can raise LDL cholesterol, multiple studies have found no consistent evidence that consuming full-fat dairy increases CVD risk. In some cases, dairy consumption has even been linked to a neutral or slightly beneficial effect on heart health. Fermented dairy products such as yogurt and cheese, especially from goats and sheep, may offer additional protection, possibly due to their probiotic content, unique fat structure, and shorter-chain saturated fats, vitamins, minerals, and bioactive compounds that may improve gut and metabolic health. Some research suggests that these products are associated with lower risks of CVD and metabolic disorders including diabetes, though the exact mechanisms are still being explored.

Goat's dairy, often consumed in the Mediterranean is generally less likely to adversely affect cholesterol levels compared to cow's dairy. Goat milk contains a higher proportion of medium-chain fatty acids (MCFAs), such as capric and caprylic acids, which are metabolized rapidly for energy rather than being stored as fat. These MCFAs have minimal impact on LDL cholesterol levels and may even have beneficial effects on metabolism. In contrast, cow dairy contains higher levels of long-chain saturated fatty acids like palmitic and myristic acids, which are more strongly associated with raising LDL cholesterol. Goat and sheep dairy also tends to have a more favorable fatty acid profile overall, with slightly higher levels of heart-friendly monounsaturated fats.

Although healthy dairy products can be enjoyed in moderation, it's important to remember that ice cream is an ultra-processed food with cream, sugar, and other added ingredients. Many cheeses used by the food industry and fast-food industry are highly processed as well. Low-fat flavored yogurts may well contain added sugars and syrups. These are not healthy products.

There are other examples where it's helpful to consider the whole food rather than to focus simply on the fat content. For example, dark chocolate is high in saturated fat, but it's often considered beneficial for health due to its high content of *flavonoids* (antioxidant polyphenol compounds found in cocoa that may support heart health). Research suggests that moderate consumption of dark chocolate can improve blood vessel function, reduce blood pressure, and have anti-inflammatory effects, which may help lower cardiovascular disease risk. The primary type of saturated fat in dark chocolate, stearic acid, has a neutral effect on LDL cholesterol. However, the health benefits depend on cocoa content, with higher percentages (70 percent or more) providing more flavonoids and less added sugar, which is a key factor in maintaining its positive effects. You can find dark chocolates of the same cocoa percentage with very different sugar amounts. If you like the pleasantly bitter taste of a healthy high cocoa chocolate, it's always a good idea to read the label and understand the sugar content and compare it with others.

Focusing on Cholesterol-Friendly Foods

Some fabulous foods actually *help* cholesterol levels. We explore them in greater depth as part of our recommended dietary patterns in Chapter 6. Here, we look at the mechanisms by which these foods have a positive effect on cholesterol.

Recognizing the importance of fiber

Fiber is a type of carbohydrate found in plant–based foods that the body can't fully digest. It plays a key role in digestion, cholesterol management, and overall health.

WARNING

When carbohydrates are refined, much of the fiber is removed during production. Refined carbohydrates can be responsible for raising cholesterol, whereas the fiber in unprocessed carbs is an important factor in reducing and controlling cholesterol.

There are two main types of fiber:

>> **Soluble:** Soluble fiber dissolves in water to form a gel-like substance that helps lower cholesterol. It's found in foods like oats, beans, and apples.

>> **Insoluble:** Insoluble fiber does not dissolve in water and mainly aids digestion. It's found in whole grains and vegetables.

Both types of fiber are important for health, but soluble fiber has the greatest impact on cholesterol levels. Soluble fiber lowers cholesterol in two key ways:

>> It interferes with the absorption of cholesterol from food.

>> It affects how the body produces cholesterol.

TECHNICAL STUFF

In Chapter 2, we explain the role of the liver in using cholesterol to make bile acids. Bile acids help digest fats. When soluble fiber binds to bile acids in the gut, it prevents them from being reabsorbed and forces the liver to use more cholesterol from the bloodstream to produce new bile acids. This process helps lower LDL cholesterol.

Soluble fiber also supports a healthy gut microbiome. When gut bacteria ferment soluble fiber, they produce short-chain fatty acids, which can enter the bloodstream and signal the liver to reduce cholesterol production. A well-balanced gut microbiome is also linked to higher levels of HDL cholesterol, which helps remove excess cholesterol from circulation (see Chapter 2).

REMEMBER

Although fiber doesn't directly bind to saturated fats, it promotes a healthier metabolism and gut environment, helping the body process fats more efficiently. The recommended daily intake of fiber is 25 to 35 grams per day.

TECHNICAL STUFF

Beta-glucan is an example of a soluble fiber found in foods like oats, barley, and certain mushrooms. The U.S. Food and Drug Administration (FDA), which regulates food labels, allows a health claim stating that 3 grams of beta-glucan per day from oats or barley can help reduce the risk of heart disease by lowering LDL cholesterol. In Europe, the scientific committee of the equivalent body has approved a claim that 3 grams of oat or barley beta-glucan daily contributes to maintaining normal blood cholesterol levels and reducing blood cholesterol, which lowers the risk of coronary heart disease. These health claims are based on strong scientific evidence showing that regular intake of beta-glucan helps lower LDL cholesterol by reducing cholesterol absorption and increasing its excretion.

Most people on a typical western diet consume only about 15 grams per day. There are several reasons why people on a western diet tend to have low fiber intakes. The western diet is often high in processed foods, which are typically low in fiber, and people in western countries tend to eat fewer fruits, vegetables, and whole grains than people in other parts of the world. The recommended dietary patterns in Chapter 6 and the delicious recipes in Chapter 15 will help you to increase the fiber in your diet.

Appreciating healthy fats and stanols

Unsaturated fats, unlike some subtypes of saturated fats, generally have a positive impact on cholesterol levels. These fats, mostly found in plant-based oils and fatty fish, tend to lower LDL cholesterol. They can also raise HDL cholesterol. As we mention earlier, there are two types of unsaturated fats:

» **Monounsaturated:** Monounsaturated fats have been shown to be particularly beneficial for heart health. They can help lower LDL cholesterol without affecting HDL cholesterol levels, or in some cases, even slightly increasing HDL. They're found in foods like olive oil, avocados, and nuts. Incorporating monounsaturated fats into your diet can be a simple yet effective way to improve your cholesterol profile.

» **Polyunsaturated:** Polyunsaturated fats include omega-3 and omega-6 fatty acids. Omega-3 fatty acids, abundant in oily fish such as salmon, mackerel, and sardines, are particularly powerful. They not only lower LDL cholesterol but also reduce triglycerides. Omega-6 fatty acids, found in vegetable oils like corn oil and safflower oil, also contribute to lowering LDL cholesterol. However, you need to maintain a balance between omega-3 and omega-6 intake, because excessive consumption of omega-6s without sufficient omega-3s may be pro-inflammatory and, for this reason, may not provide the same heart-protective benefits. Focusing on incorporating sustainable oily fish into your diet at least twice a week and regularly choosing many of the green leafy vegetables, which also contain omega-3s, is a great way to boost your omega-3 intake.

TIP

Replacing saturated and trans fats with unsaturated fats is a key dietary strategy for managing cholesterol levels. Many of the plant sources of unsaturated fats also contain other compounds that are important in reducing oxidation and inflammation of cholesterol.

Other types of fats in the diet can affect cholesterol levels, too. Fats called *stanols* are a type of plant *sterol*, which are compounds found in plants that are structurally similar to cholesterol and can help reduce its absorption and found in small amounts in foods like whole grains, nuts, seeds, legumes, fruits, and vegetables. They're structurally similar to cholesterol, and they work by blocking cholesterol absorption in the intestines, leading to lower LDL cholesterol levels without affecting HDL cholesterol. Stanols and sterols are collectively called *phytosterols*. (*Phyto-* simply means "of plant origin.")

Powering up with protein

Of the three macronutrients — fat, carbohydrate, and protein — protein has the least direct effect on cholesterol. However, when people eat meals, they generally incorporate all three macronutrients. Even though people often categorize a food by its most common macronutrient, whole foods are often made up of more than one macronutrient. Because fats and carbohydrates affect cholesterol levels, when you think of the protein in your diet, be sure to consider any fats and carbohydrates that are co-ingredients in protein-dominant foods.

For example, as a protein source, red meat also contains saturated fat, which raises cholesterol levels. Fish, on the other hand, is a protein-rich food with omega-3 unsaturated fats, which have the opposite effect. Protein in nuts is accompanied by beneficial monounsaturated fats. One of the healthiest protein choices you can make is to enjoy beans, which deliver high quantities of cholesterol-reducing fiber.

TIP

Plant-based protein foods often contain other nutrients that help cholesterol levels and support a healthy gut microbiome.

Getting the right vitamins and minerals

The carbohydrates, fats, and proteins that provide the energy and chemical building blocks for life are known as *macronutrients*, because they're the nutrients consumed in the greatest amount. Minerals and vitamins — called *micronutrients* — are needed in smaller amounts but they're also essential for the many processes that maintain health.

Several vitamins and minerals directly influence cholesterol levels and contribute to cholesterol regulation:

>> **Niacin (vitamin B3):** Niacin is one of the most well-documented nutrients for cholesterol management. It can increase HDL cholesterol while lowering LDL cholesterol and triglycerides. However, in order for these effects to be seen, high doses are required, generally more than the amounts in a typical diet, even one rich in the meat, fish, vegetables, beans, and whole grains that contain niacin. Therapeutic niacin supplements to lower cholesterol should only be taken under medical supervision.

>> **Vitamin C and E:** These vitamins have antioxidant effects. They may reduce levels of oxidative stress and contribute to the reduced oxidation of LDL cholesterol.

- >> **Vitamin D:** Vitamin D may also play a role in cholesterol metabolism, because low levels have been linked to higher LDL cholesterol and lower HDL cholesterol, though more research is needed to confirm its direct impact.

- >> **Magnesium:** Magnesium has been associated with lower LDL and higher HDL cholesterol, potentially improving cholesterol balance.

- >> **Zinc:** Zinc may help regulate lipid metabolism and maintain balanced cholesterol levels.

- >> **Selenium:** Selenium plays a role in preventing LDL oxidation.

- >> **Calcium:** Calcium, when consumed in adequate amounts, may also help reduce LDL cholesterol.

REMEMBER

Vitamins and minerals are often sold in supplements. For most people, there is no evidence that consuming amounts greater than those found in a healthy diet is beneficial for cholesterol and cardiovascular health unless your physician has specifically recommended them for a deficiency or specific medical reason. A possible exception to this may be vitamin D — many people, especially in temperate climates, don't make enough vitamin D because they don't get enough exposure to sunlight.

Talk to your healthcare provider if you're considering taking a supplement.

Managing oxidative stress with polyphenols

There is increasing research showing the importance of bioactive compounds for protection against numerous chronic diseases, often because they prevent the potentially damaging and disrupting effects of oxidation and inflammation (see Chapter 4).

Bioactive compounds are naturally occurring substances found in small quantities in various foods, including fruits, vegetables, whole grains, and even some beverages like tea and wine. Some prominent subgroups of bioactive compounds include *polyphenols* (such as flavonoids and anthocyanins, known for their antioxidant properties), *carotenoids* (like beta-carotene and lycopene, often associated with vision and immune health), and *organosulfur* compounds (found in garlic and onions, which may have anti-inflammatory and anti-cancer effects). Research continues to explore the specific mechanisms by which these compounds exert their beneficial effects and the optimal dietary intakes for maximizing their potential, but we know they have an important role to play in human health.

Polyphenols, of which more than 8,000 have been identified so far, are produced by plants to counteract harmful oxidation reactions in their environment similar to those illustrated in Chapter 4. They protect plants from UV light and radiation, and many have antimicrobial effects — resisting infections and infestations that could damage the plant or its fruit.

TECHNICAL STUFF

Some polyphenols in fruits are brightly colored. (Changes in polyphenol color in the fruit can signify to animals or birds when they're ready to be eaten, by which time the seed has matured.) Alternatively, many polyphenols have a pungent or bitter taste to protect parts of the plant from being eaten or fruits consumed too early, before the seed is ready.

TIP

A report published based on analysis of the results of the respected Predimed (Prevención con Dieta Mediterránea) study in Spain found that those who reported eating diets rich in polyphenols had a 46 percent lower risk of developing heart disease than those who ate the least. This is an extraordinary discovery and may well be directly related to the ability of polyphenols in the diet to reduce oxidation of LDL cholesterol and inflammation of cholesterol-generated atherosclerotic plaques.

Grasping the role of the gut microbiome

The gut is home to trillions of tiny organisms, including bacteria, fungi, and viruses, collectively known as the *gut microbiome*. When this community is balanced and diverse, it plays a vital role in digestion, nutrient absorption, immune function, and even mental health. However, when the gut microbiome becomes imbalanced — a condition called *dysbiosis* — it can contribute to various health issues, including obesity, diabetes, and heart disease.

One of the gut microbiome's key roles is helping to regulate cholesterol levels, which is crucial for heart health. Some beneficial gut bacteria help lower cholesterol by breaking it down or preventing it from being absorbed into the bloodstream. Others convert cholesterol into a substance called *coprostanol,* which the body can't absorb, so it simply passes through. This natural process helps keep cholesterol levels in check.

However, an unhealthy gut microbiome can have the opposite effect. Some harmful bacteria produce substances that encourage the liver to make more cholesterol or increase how much cholesterol the body absorbs from food. This can raise cholesterol levels and increase the risk of cardiovascular disease. That's why maintaining a healthy gut is so important for heart health.

Eating a diet rich in plant-based foods can help nourish beneficial gut bacteria. The Mediterranean diet is renowned for many health benefits, including maintaining a healthy microbiome due to the high fiber content, including the presence of key *prebiotics* (nondigestible food ingredients that promote the growth of beneficial bacteria) and *probiotics* (live microorganisms that, when consumed in adequate amounts, add to and support the microbiome). Polyphenols can also be considered as food for these bacteria, helping them grow and thrive. By feeding good bacteria, polyphenols support a diverse microbiome that is better equipped to manage cholesterol and keep inflammation in check. Interestingly, gut bacteria also help unlock the full potential of polyphenols. When we consume polyphenol-rich foods, our gut microbes break them down into smaller compounds that have even stronger antioxidant and anti-inflammatory effects, protecting blood vessels, reducing inflammation, and lowering the risk of CVD.

Chapter **6**

Discovering the Best Diet for Cholesterol Management

n order for us to recommend a diet for cholesterol management, it must have some key characteristics. There must be convincing scientific evidence to confirm that the diet will

» **Improve cholesterol levels.** It must contain foods that improve your cholesterol ratio by decreasing low-density lipoprotein (LDL) cholesterol and increasing high-density lipoprotein (HDL) cholesterol. It must also reduce oxidation and inflammation through foods rich in bioactive compounds like polyphenols.

» **Reduce the risk of atherosclerosis, heart disease and stroke.** It must not only be able to improve cholesterol results and be known to reduce oxidative stress and oxidized LDL (see Chapter 4), but also lead to reduced rates of plaque formation, atherosclerosis, and cardiovascular diseases (CVDs). In other words, the diet must be protective from the conditions associated with high cholesterol.

>> **Improve health and well-being in general.** It must reduce other chronic diseases, including cancer, dementia, and diabetes; improve mental and physical health; and support optimum weight. There is little point in following a diet in the hopes of reducing cholesterol levels if it lacks essential nutrients or increases your risk of other diseases like cancer and diabetes.

>> **Be sustainable for you individually.** Many diets are not enjoyable and are unable to be maintained for long periods of time. Managing cholesterol is a lifelong commitment, so a diet that you have to follow for life needs to be *very* enjoyable, affordable, and compatible with a healthy overall lifestyle.

>> **Be sustainable for the environment.** What's good for you as an individual must also be good for the planet. Food production currently makes a significant contribution to carbon emissions, but we can make an impact on that with a diet that's more environmentally friendly.

The dietary pattern that fulfills all these criteria is — drumroll, please — the Mediterranean diet. In 2025, the Mediterranean diet was named the best overall diet for the eighth year in a row by a committee of respected nutrition experts commissioned to assess different diets by *U.S. News & World Report.* The diet also gained the prestigious top spot for best diets for cholesterol management, diabetes, mental health, and gut health. This evidence-based assessment reflects the significant amount of published peer-reviewed research.

We've been advocates of the Mediterranean diet for many years, publishing numerous books and articles on the subject. Amy's recipes in Chapter 15 are all aligned with the Mediterranean diet and lifestyle.

In this chapter, we walk through what the Mediterranean diet is and the benefits it offers.

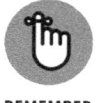

REMEMBER

The word *diet* actually derives from the ancient Greek word *diaita,* which means "way of living," and it's liberating to think of enjoying foods in that spirit.

Defining the Mediterranean Diet

The Mediterranean diet conforms to the true meaning of the Greek word *diaita.* It's a way of life with culinary traditions deeply rooted in the history and culture of the Mediterranean region. Its origins can be traced back to the ancient civilizations that flourished around the Mediterranean Basin, including Greece, Italy, Spain, the Levant (the eastern Mediterranean), and North Africa. These cultures shared a common approach to both lifestyle and food, emphasizing fresh, seasonal produce; lean proteins; and healthy fats.

The Mediterranean diet is characterized by a rich tapestry of flavors and ingredients, reflecting the diverse culinary traditions of the region. It has evolved over time, with trade introducing new elements, including many herbs and spices from Asia; coffee from Africa; and tomatoes, corn, peppers, potatoes, and chocolate from the Americas.

At its core, the Mediterranean diet is a foundation of plant-based foods, including an abundance of vegetables, fruits, whole grains, legumes, nuts, and seeds. These foods provide essential vitamins, minerals, antioxidants, and fiber, contributing to overall health and well-being, as well as cholesterol management.

Olive oil is the cornerstone of the Mediterranean diet, serving as the primary source of added fat. Rich in monounsaturated fats, olive oil has been linked to numerous health benefits, including reducing the risk of heart disease and stroke. Other healthy fats, such as those found in avocados, nuts, and seeds, are also incorporated into the diet.

Although plant-based foods take center stage, the Mediterranean diet also includes moderate amounts of fish and poultry. These protein sources provide essential nutrients without the high saturated fat content found in red meat, which is eaten less frequently, typically only a few times per month. Dairy, especially fermented foods like yogurt and cheese, are consumed in moderate amounts, especially sourced from the milk of goats and sheep.

Sweets and desserts are enjoyed occasionally as treats, and added sugars are from natural products such as honey. Ultra-processed foods with ingredients like trans fats and emulsifiers are excluded entirely and have no place in the diet.

Figure 6-1 shows the Mediterranean Diet Pyramid from Oldways, an organization offering education on "shared cultural food traditions from around the world."

The Mediterranean diet is completely aligned with the macronutrients, micronutrients and bioactive compounds found in foods that benefit cholesterol, either directly or indirectly through a healthy gut microbiome (see Chapter 5). As a lifestyle, there is emphasis on balance, moderation, and enjoyment of meals. Meals are often shared with family and friends, fostering a sense of community and connection. Physical activity is also an integral part of the Mediterranean lifestyle, as well as strategies to maximize well-being, which may, through a reduction in stress hormones such as cortisol, improve cholesterol profile. We explore these subjects in greater detail in Chapters 9, 10, and 12.

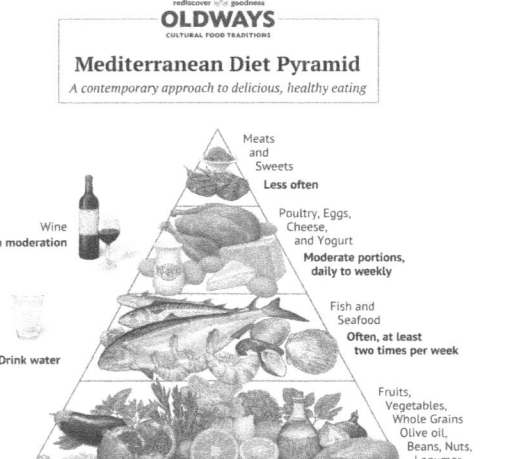

FIGURE 6-1:
The
Mediterranean
Diet Pyramid.

Comparing the Mediterranean Diet to the Western Diet

Unfortunately, the standard Western diet is a long way from the traditional Mediterranean diet outlined in the preceding section. Tables 6-1, 6-2, and 6-3 paint the picture.

TABLE 6-1   **The Western Diet versus the Mediterranean Diet: Macronutrient Composition**

Macronutrient	Western Diet	Mediterranean Diet
Fats	35%–45% (mostly saturated and trans fats)	30%–40% (mostly monounsaturated and polyunsaturated fats)
Carbohydrates	45%–50% (refined, processed carbs)	45%–55% (whole grains, legumes, fruits, and vegetables)
Proteins	15%–20% (mostly red meats and processed meats)	10%–15% (mostly plant-based proteins and fish)

TABLE 6-2 The Western Diet versus the Mediterranean Diet: Key Food Type Consumption

Food Type	Western Diet	Mediterranean Diet
Vegetables and fruits	About 3 servings per day	7–10 servings per day
Whole grains	15%–20% of grain intake	50%–60% of grain intake
Red meat and processed meat	About 110–150 grams per day	About 20–50 grams per week
Fish and seafood	Less than 1 serving per week	2–4 servings per week
Legumes	About 1 serving per week	About 4–7 servings per week
Dairy	High (processed cheese, butter)	Moderate (yogurt, cheese)
Nuts and seeds	Less than 1 serving/week	About 1 serving per day
Olive oil	Minimal use	Primary fat source (about 2–3 tablespoons or 25–50 milliliters per day)
Added sugars	About 15%–20% of daily energy intake	Less than 5% of daily energy intake
Ultra-processed foods	About 50%–60% of total calories	Less than 10% of total calories

TABLE 6-3 The Western Diet versus the Mediterranean Diet: Health Impact

Health Metric	Western Diet	Mediterranean Diet
Obesity rate	36% (United States), 20%–30% (Europe)	10%–15% (Mediterranean regions)
CVD risk	High (leading cause of death)	30% lower risk
Type 2 diabetes risk	2–4 times higher risk than Mediterranean diet	52% reduced risk
Life expectancy	About 78 years (United States)	About 83 years (Mediterranean countries)

In 2019, researchers published a modeling study in the *Food and Nutrition Journal* in which they estimated healthcare savings due to reductions in CVD incidence if a higher percentage of the population adopted a more Mediterranean dietary pattern. An increasing percentage of population adhering to a Mediterranean diet by 20 percent beyond the current adherence level could produce annual savings in CVD-related costs of US$8.2 billion in the United States and C$320 million in Canada. An 80 percent increase in adherence resulted in savings equal to US$31 billion in the United States and C$1.2 billion in Canada, according to the modeling.

FATS AND CALORIES

You may concerned about eating foods that contain fat because you've heard the over-simplistic advice to reduce the amount of fat in your diet. Or perhaps you thought the term *dietary fat* implies that eating it will make you fat.

The Mediterranean diet is not particularly low in fat, but the fats are healthy fats that improve cholesterol levels. It's also a diet where food choices are more important than counting calories.

There is good evidence that the monounsaturated fats in olive oil help to stimulate body fat breakdown and inhibit body fat production. A diet rich in monounsaturated fats may modify the body composition of obese individuals by increasing their lean body mass and decreasing the percentage of body fat.

Most health professionals now recognize that the different types of fats in foods have different effects not only on cholesterol but also on the likelihood of your putting on extra weight.

Among the three macronutrients, fats contain the most calories. The calorie content of a food is the amount of energy a food can provide. Excess calories in the diet may result in that energy being stored as body fat. However, it's a bit more complicated than that. Our bodies don't simply add up the calories consumed, subtract the energy used, and put the difference onto our waistlines.

Calories from different sources can affect the body's hormonal balance and energy usage differently, influencing hunger, satiety, and overall metabolic health. For example, fat from olive oil helps to reduce the speed of sugar absorption from carbohydrates and makes the hormone insulin more sensitive to the rise in blood glucose following a meal. Calories from the sugars in refined carbohydrates can be more likely to result in weight gain than calories from dietary fat.

Understanding what *overweight* truly means is also key. Your doctor may determine your body mass index (BMI) using a height and weight calculation. This BMI categorizes you as underweight, normal weight, overweight, or obese. In Western societies, the combination of a typical diet and lack of exercise makes being overweight or obese a risk factor for conditions like diabetes, cardiovascular disease, and some cancers.

BMI calculations, while useful, have some drawbacks when it comes to assessing health risks. For example, they can't differentiate between excess body fat and greater muscle mass. A professional athlete, like an American football player or an Australian rugby player, may have a high BMI due to their muscle mass, not excess fat.

Bone density and lean muscle also contribute to weight, and these are important, especially for older adults, for maintaining strength and reducing fracture risk. Furthermore, BMI alone doesn't tell the whole story about health risks. A healthy diet and lifestyle can lessen the increased risk of health problems associated with being overweight.

A 2020 study from Uppsala University in Sweden, involving 79,000 participants over 21 years, illustrates this point. Researchers tracked both BMI and adherence to a Mediterranean diet. They discovered that overweight individuals who closely followed a Mediterranean diet had the lowest risk of death from any cause. Obese individuals eating this diet didn't have a higher overall mortality risk but did show an increased risk of heart disease. Interestingly, even those at a healthy weight but with poor adherence to a Mediterranean diet had higher mortality rates than those at the same weight who regularly consumed such a diet.

If you're overweight, adopting a Mediterranean-style diet, rich in olive oil (even though it contains healthy fats), can be a helpful step toward achieving a healthier weight. Prioritizing a nutritious diet is crucial for minimizing the risks of diabetes, heart disease, cancers, and chronic inflammation, all of which can be linked to being overweight while following a Western diet.

Weighing the Evidence for the Mediterranean Diet

The Mediterranean diet was first identified by U.S. physician and professor Ancel Keys and his colleagues, who studied the traditional dietary patterns that had been followed for thousands of years. In the 1950s and 1960s, Keys observed communities in Southern Italy and Greece and noted that their way of eating seemed to provide significant protection against chronic diseases. At the same time, conditions like heart disease, stroke, and diabetes were becoming increasingly common in the United States and Northern Europe.

Since then, extensive research has repeatedly confirmed that the Mediterranean diet is strongly linked to a lower risk of numerous health conditions, including heart disease, stroke, diabetes, obesity, high blood pressure, several forms of cancer, arthritis and other inflammatory disorders, Alzheimer's disease, Parkinson's disease, vascular dementia, depression, and even premature death.

One of the most frequently cited studies on the Mediterranean diet is the PREDIMED study (Prevención con Dieta Mediterránea). Conducted in Spain, this randomized controlled trial followed 7,447 individuals ages 55 to 80, all of whom were at high cardiovascular risk but had no diagnosed disease. Participants were monitored for five years, following either a Mediterranean diet enriched with extra-virgin olive oil or nuts or a conventional low-fat diet. The study found that those on the Mediterranean diet experienced a more than 30 percent reduction in heart attack, stroke, or death from cardiovascular causes. Additionally, in a subset of the study, there was a 40 percent lower risk of developing type 2 diabetes and a 68 percent reduction in breast cancer incidence. Significant reductions in cognitive decline, dementia, and other chronic conditions were also observed.

Adopting a Mediterranean-style diet has been shown to enhance blood vessel function and even reverse early-stage atherosclerosis. It's also associated with a lower risk of erectile dysfunction and improved sexual health overall. The advantages can begin almost immediately, with noticeable improvements in some health markers within weeks, and benefits can still be achieved even when changes are made later in life. Importantly, the Mediterranean diet's effectiveness is not limited to Mediterranean populations. Studies across different ethnic groups and regions worldwide have demonstrated its powerful health benefits well beyond its place of origin.

The PREDIMED trial found that people following a Mediterranean diet supplemented with either olive oil or nuts experienced improvements in their cholesterol profiles, including lower levels of LDL cholesterol and triglycerides, and higher levels of HDL cholesterol.

The researchers involved in the PREDIMED study also looked at a smaller group of people participating in the project and used ultrasound techniques to look at plaques and the rate of progression in the *carotid artery* (the blood vessel supplying the brain). They found that there was a significant reduction in the thickness and growth of plaques with the Mediterranean diet. This was consistent with the overall study results, which showed a 30 percent reduction in risk of strokes.

Other research has looked at the direct impact of the Mediterranean diet on the arteries themselves. The CORDIOPREV study, a randomized controlled trial that followed patients with existing heart disease, showed that a Mediterranean diet rich in olive oil helped to slow down the progression of atherosclerosis. They measured this by looking at the thickness of the artery walls and characteristics of the plaques themselves. Similarly, the ILERVAS cohort study from Spain found that people who closely followed a Mediterranean diet were less likely to develop plaque in their arteries in the first place.

Ongoing research, like the MEDIMACS trial, based in numerous centers and looking at patients with acute coronary syndrome, who present with sudden symptoms of heart atherosclerosis, is delving even deeper into how the Mediterranean diet affects plaque stability. Unstable plaques are more prone to rupture, which can trigger a heart attack or stroke, and early data is suggesting that the Mediterranean diet improves stability. This research is looking at many aspects including inflammation and the gut microbiome.

Certain Mediterranean regions have become renowned for showcasing the benefits of this lifestyle. The Greek island of Crete and the region of Calabria in Southern Italy were both part of Ancel Keys's Seven Countries Study, while Sardinia and Ikaria have gained recognition for their exceptionally high number of centenarians — remarkable even within the Mediterranean. Ikaria, in particular, stands out: Residents live an average of eight to ten years longer than their counterparts in the United States. The likelihood of reaching 90 is twice as high for Ikarians, and one in three people surpasses that milestone. Their quality of life remains excellent, with lower rates of chronic illness, preserved cognitive health, and strong community engagement. More than 80 percent of those over 65 report having an active and fulfilling sex life. This specific finding may relate to lower levels of atherosclerosis in blood vessels supplying sexual organs.

Making the Mediterranean Diet Work for You

In Chapter 5, we cover the nutrients in foods that affect circulating cholesterol levels — from its absorption and its production, regulation, and transport, to the chemical processes of oxidation and inflammation, which make it more dangerous. In this section, we dive deeper and look at the actual foods that are common in the Mediterranean diet and that you can add to your pantry, use in your cooking, and rely on as the most delicious basis for your meals.

Incorporating the foods that lower cholesterol

Meals should be a combination of healthy fats, proteins, and carbohydrates. Here are foods you should try to include each day:

>> **Whole grains:** Whole grains are rich in soluble fiber, which binds to cholesterol in the digestive tract, reducing its absorption and lowering LDL cholesterol. Studies show that regular consumption of whole grains lowers LDL cholesterol. Complex carbohydrates digest slowly with a low glycemic index (GI), preventing insulin spikes that can contribute to poor cholesterol regulation known as *dyslipidemia* and potentially lead to weight gain and type 2 diabetes. Examples of whole grains include amaranth, barley, brown rice, buckwheat, bulgur, farro, freekeh, millet, quinoa, rye, sorghum, teff, whole-grain couscous, whole-grain pasta, and whole-wheat bread.

» **Vegetables:** Many vegetables are high in fiber, helping lower cholesterol by promoting its excretion, and are low GI. Many vegetables also contain bioactive compounds like carotenoids and polyphenols that protect LDL from oxidation. Examples of vegetables that help lower cholesterol include cruciferous vegetables (broccoli, Brussels sprouts, cabbage, cauliflower), leafy greens (arugula, collard greens, kale, lettuce, spinach, Swiss chard), nightshades (eggplant, peppers, tomatoes, zucchini), root vegetables (beets, carrots, radishes, sweet potatoes), and other Mediterranean staples like artichokes, asparagus, fennel, leeks, and onions.

» **Whole fruits:** Fiber in the whole fruit not only reduces cholesterol absorption, but "locks" the sugars into the *food matrix* (the food's physical structure), resulting in slow absorption, a low GI, and less likelihood of glucose- and insulin-related dyslipidemia. Fruits are also rich in antioxidant bioactive compounds. Examples include apples, apricots, berries (blackberries, blueberries, raspberries, strawberries), cherries, dates, figs, grapefruits, grapes, kiwis, lemons, limes, melons (cantaloupe, honeydew, watermelon), nectarines, oranges, peaches, pears, plums, and pomegranates.

» **Nuts and seeds:** Nuts and seeds are high in monounsaturated and polyunsaturated fats that help lower LDL cholesterol. Many contain plant sterols that naturally block cholesterol absorption from the gut. They're a rich source of vitamins and minerals that may support healthy cholesterol levels, as well as bioactive compounds that reduce the risk of oxidation of LDL. Examples include almonds, Brazil nuts, cashews, chia seeds, flaxseeds, hazelnuts, hemp seeds, pecans, pine nuts, pistachios, pumpkin seeds, sesame seeds, sunflower seeds, and walnuts.

» **Legumes:** Legumes are an excellent source of soluble fiber and are a good protein alternative to meat, with little or no saturated fat. They're also rich in vitamins, minerals, and bioactive compounds. Examples include beans (black, cannellini, lima, kidney, navy, pinto, white, fava, soybeans/edamame), chickpeas, lentils (black, brown, green, red), peas, and lupins.

» **Extra-virgin olive oil:** Extra-virgin olive oil is high in the monounsaturated fat oleic acid, which helps to lower LDL cholesterol while maintaining HDL cholesterol. Many extra-virgin olive oils contain high quantities of polyphenols, which prevent oxidation of LDL cholesterol. There are many different varieties of extra-virgin olive oil, a ubiquitous ingredient in the Mediterranean diet. (For more on extra-virgin olive oil, see the nearby sidebar.)

» **Fish and seafood:** Oily fish are rich in omega-3 fatty acids, which lower triglycerides and increase HDL cholesterol, in addition to having anti-inflammatory properties. Examples include fatty fish (herring, mackerel, salmon, sardines, trout, tuna), octopus, shellfish (clams, mussels, oysters, scallops, shrimp), squid, and whitefish (cod, haddock, sea bass, snapper, sole).

THE SPECIAL ROLE OF EXTRA-VIRGIN OLIVE OIL

Research shows that the more closely people follow a Mediterranean diet rich in extra-virgin olive oil, the better their cholesterol profile, the lower the amount of circulating oxidized cholesterol and biomarkers of inflammation, and the lower their risk of cardiovascular disease.

Extra-virgin olive oil is at the heart of the Mediterranean diet, used in cooking and adding flavor and nutrition. There is no single ingredient that contributes so much to any diet in the world. In many parts of the Mediterranean, olive trees stretch as far as the eye can see, and the oil they produce has been enjoyed and celebrated for millennia as the main source of dietary fat, frequently making up as much as 20 percent to 30 percent of total calories.

Landmark studies have shown the extraordinary effects of extra-virgin olive oil:

- A study conducted in Bordeaux and published in 2011 in the journal *Neurology* showed a 41 percent difference in the risk of stroke between the lowest and highest extra-virgin olive oil consumers.

- In 2012, the multicenter EPIC study (The European Prospective Investigation into Cancer and Nutrition), observed that the risk of developing heart disease was halved by the regular consumption of extra-virgin olive oil.

- In 2013, the PREDIMED study showed that heart disease, stroke, and overall deaths were reduced by a third in people consuming the Mediterranean diet supplemented with extra-virgin olive oil.

In 2023, a review of the established evidence was published in the journal *Nutrients* with the title "Is Extra-Virgin Olive Oil the Critical Ingredient Driving the Health Benefits of a Mediterranean Diet? A Narrative Review." The article discussed the benefits of the monounsaturated fat oleic acid found in olive oil, which has cholesterol-lowering and anti-inflammatory effects. The authors also concluded that the antioxidant and anti-inflammatory effects of key polyphenols in extra-virgin olive oil are probably even more important, especially in reducing oxidation of LDL cholesterol.

The U.S. Food and Drug Administration (FDA) and the European Food Safety Authority (EFSA) allow producers of olive oil to state on their labels the benefits of the monounsaturated fats in olive oil in reducing LDL cholesterol and CVD.

(continued)

(continued)

EFSA has also authorized producers of extra-virgin olive oil with a particular level of polyphenols to state that "olive oil polyphenols contribute to the protection of blood lipids from oxidative stress." This is based on evidence that if you consume a certain amount (more than 1½ tablespoons or 20 milliliters per day) of an extra-virgin olive oil that contains a particular minimum level of polyphenols, there will be a measurable effect on oxidized LDL cholesterol.

Cooking, including frying, at all usual temperatures with extra-virgin olive oil, as they do in the Mediterranean diet, is safe and beneficial. The high monounsaturated fat content and polyphenol antioxidants in extra-virgin olive oil make it more resistant to breaking down and forming harmful compounds, including trans fats, at high temperatures compared to other cooking oils, especially those high in polyunsaturated fats. Some polyphenols in extra-virgin olive oil may be lost during cooking, but studies show that significant amounts remain, and they even transfer to the food being cooked, increasing its antioxidant content.

Our book *Olive Oil For Dummies* (published by John Wiley & Sons, Inc.) tells you everything you need to know about olive oil, its health and culinary benefits, how to choose the best extra-virgin olive oil, and how to get the best value for your money. Not all extra-virgin olive oils are the same, and most don't have sufficiently high levels of polyphenols to meet the European claim for reducing oxidized LDL. Olives of particular varieties, nurtured, harvested early, pressed in controlled conditions soon after picking, and stored away from heat, light, and oxygen are needed to ensure the minimum levels of polyphenols.

You can recognize an extra-virgin olive oil that's rich in polyphenols because it has a pleasant bitterness and pungency in its flavor profile. In Europe, you may see an EFSA-authorized health claim on the label of the bottle to support a high-polyphenol description.

>> **Poultry:** Poultry provides protein and many essential nutrients with less saturated fat than red meat. Examples include chicken, duck. game birds (partridge, pheasant, quail), and turkey.

>> **Dairy:** Despite the presence of saturated fat, the short- and medium-chain subtypes, especially common in goat and sheep milk in the Mediterranean may not have an adverse effect of other saturated fats. The probiotics in yogurt and cheese (fermented milk) may also help improve cholesterol levels by supporting gut health (see Chapter 5). Examples include cheese (feta,

halloumi, Manchego, mozzarella, Parmesan, pecorino, ricotta), milk (cow, goat, sheep), and yogurt (goat, Greek, plain, sheep).

>> **Red wine:** A small amount of red wine may reduce LDL cholesterol, improve HDL cholesterol, and reduce LDL oxidation with polyphenols such as procyanidins and resveratrol. Examples include Mediterranean red wines such as Chianti (Italy), Rioja (Spain), Bordeaux (France), Agiorgitiko (Greece), and Tempranillo (Spain). There are particular red wine varieties rich in polyphenols, such as Madiran from southwestern France, Barolo from the Piedmont region of Italy, and Cannonau from Sardinia.

Reducing oxidative stress and inflammation

In Chapter 4, we cover oxidation, oxidative stress, chronic inflammation, and the role these play in forming damaging oxidized LDL cholesterol and atherosclerotic plaques. Important plant compounds known as *polyphenols* have the capacity to prevent and protect us from these processes (see Chapter 5). The way our bodies handle polyphenols in the diet and their antioxidant and anti-inflammatory effects are not yet fully understood. Scientists dedicate conferences to debating what's known and unknown, but few doubt the significance of polyphenols. What is clear is that supplements are not the answer — there is very little evidence that taking polyphenol extracts in pills does any good, probably because the way polyphenols in food are metabolized and altered by our individual gut microbiomes is key.

TECHNICAL
STUFF

Scientists are not yet entirely clear exactly how polyphenols work in the body, and to what extent this varies between individuals. The chemistry of polyphenols is altered by gut microbes, so it may be that the products of these compounds are what's most active. Antioxidant processes in laboratory test tube experiments — so-called *in vitro* investigations — are different from the effects observed *in vivo*, with animal or human studies. Measuring oxidation of LDL cholesterol in real-time experiments is challenging, which is why it isn't (yet) used routinely as a clinical test. This is a fascinating area of work, and it's opening up a new understanding of the oxidation of cholesterol and inflammation.

Several different types of polyphenols and subgroups — called *flavonoids* — are of particular interest to scientists because of their potential to improve cholesterol profiles and reduce oxidized LDL and inflammation. Here are some notable examples of foods high in flavonoids. (This list is not exhaustive — it just illustrates the range of flavonoid polyphenols and some examples of foods where they can be found.)

» **Fruits** like blackberries, blueberries, raspberries, and strawberries are high in *anthocyanins,* a type of flavonoid known to reduce LDL oxidation and inflammation. Apples, especially in the outer skin, are also a rich source of quercetin and other flavonoids. Citrus fruits like grapefruits, lemons, limes, and oranges contain flavanones like hesperidin, which are known for their protective effects against LDL oxidation. Red grapes are rich in procyanidins, resveratrol, and other flavonoids, which help reduce LDL oxidation and inflammation. Tomatoes, which are actually a type of fruit, contain flavonoids like quercetin and naringenin, in addition to lycopene, which is a carotenoid compound with antioxidant activities.

» **Vegetables:** Most vegetables, including beans and other legumes, are rich in polyphenols, especially in their colorful outer layers. For example, leafy greens like kale and spinach are packed with flavonoids like kaempferol and quercetin, which support cardiovascular health by reducing oxidative stress. Onions are high in quercetin, also protecting LDL particles from oxidation. Soy, a common ingredient in traditional Asian diets, is rich in isoflavones, which help improve cholesterol levels and prevent LDL oxidation. Luteolin is a flavonoid found in artichokes, carrots, celery, parsley, and peppers. Many purple vegetables contain anthocyanin flavonoids.

» **Herbs and spices:** Herbs and spices are an excellent source of polyphenols, including many types of flavonoids, which reduce oxidative stress and the oxidation of LDL cholesterol. With their aromatic, pungent, and sometimes bitter flavors, they're perfect to add in small quantities to foods to spice up your meals or to make refreshing herbal teas. Chili, cinnamon, cloves, ginger, oregano, pepper, rosemary, thyme, and turmeric are all examples of concentrated, polyphenol-rich herbs and spices, many of which are included in the recipes later in this book.

» **Tea and coffee:** Green tea is especially rich in catechins, while black tea has theaflavins. Both these types of flavonoids have been shown to improve lipid profiles and reduce oxidized LDL cholesterol. Coffee contains many flavonoids and also chlorogenic acids, which are polyphenols that appear to have a strong capacity to reduce LDL oxidation.

» **Dark chocolate:** Flavonoids in dark chocolate, particularly epicatechin, are associated with lower LDL cholesterol levels and reduced oxidation. Aim for chocolate with at least 70 percent cocoa content or even higher for the best benefits.

TIP

Many of these plant foods contain numerous other nutrients and bioactive compounds, including vitamin E, vitamin C, other polyphenols, and carotenoids.

Oxidative stress and chronic inflammation are linked and are closely involved in the development of atherosclerosis. Scientists can now measure signs of oxidative stress and low-grade inflammation with highly sensitive methods that can analyze and quantify chemicals that increase alongside inflammation — so called *biomarkers*. Researchers using very accurate and specialized laboratory techniques have just begun to make important discoveries about the factors in our environment and lifestyle that lead to chronic inflammation. This is resulting in some remarkable conclusions.

A low-quality diet is linked to much higher biomarkers of inflammation and risk of CVD than the Mediterranean diet does. What's quite astonishing is the speed at which changes can occur. Studies have shown that a single meal of, for example a recipe called *sofrito* (olive oil, onions, garlic, tomatoes, and herbs) can, within a matter of hours, reduce biomarkers of LDL cholesterol oxidation and inflammation. This means that what you eat *today* may have an effect on what's going on in your body to protect you from oxidative stress and plaque inflammation. This finding has challenged the historic assumptions that we describe in Chapter 1, making it clear that atherosclerosis is *not* simply a buildup in blood vessels of clogging and blocking cholesterol over many misspent years. We can conclude from the latest evidence that protection from the processes of plaque formation and instability can be influenced by a person's lifestyle *right now*. This is why it's possible to make changes at *any* stage in life to reduce the risk of plaque rupture, reduce the oxidation of LDL cholesterol, and reduce the inflammatory pathways that lead to atherosclerotic events like heart attacks and strokes.

REMEMBER

It's never too late to improve and benefit from a healthy lifestyle, full of the delicious foods that lower cholesterol and reduce oxidative stress and inflammation.

TIP

A diet high in polyphenols has been shown to reduce the risk of developing heart disease by 46 percent, but it's important to remember that this is based on consuming a healthy and balanced Mediterranean diet rich in colored vegetables, fruits, extra-virgin olive oil, nuts, herbs, and spices. There is no evidence to suggest that polyphenols in supplements can benefit health. In fact, doses in supplements may be too high and even cause harm. So, choose the kinds of foods recommended in this book and look for those naturally high in polyphenols (for example, a high-polyphenol extra-virgin olive oil.)

Studies showing reductions in heart attacks and strokes can take several years to show results, simply because it takes time to gather the required statistical numbers of these events. However, the actual changes in the body of an individual on a high-quality diet are happening in the short term as well as the long term. And this isn't just true for cholesterol, atherosclerosis, and CVD. Earlier in this chapter, we emphasize the importance of protection from other conditions and illnesses, too. The diet's anti-inflammatory properties and immune-supporting components also contribute to better outcomes in people facing acute infections, such as COVID-19.

AFFORDABILITY AND SUSTAINABILITY

There is a widespread misconception that following the Mediterranean diet outside of the region is expensive, but research from Rhode Island and separately in Australia confirmed that at least $30 per week can be shaved off grocery costs when Mediterranean diet ingredients replace a standard American food profile. This is because the Mediterranean diet is plant based and, for example, vegetables and legumes can be produced more cheaply than meats. Cooking from scratch is also a less expensive way to prepare food than to have a ready meal option.

Outside the Mediterranean region, many people have grown up with the idea that a cooking oil in a plastic bottle should be one of the cheapest items in our shopping basket. If you recognize that a good-quality extra-virgin olive oil is the foundation of the Mediterranean diet that makes affordable vegetables and legumes much more palatable and tastier, improves cholesterol, and reduces oxidative stress, it makes sense to invest a higher proportion of your weekly budget in it.

The sustainability credentials of the Mediterranean diet are well established. Its emphasis on plant-based foods, like fruits, vegetables, grains, and legumes, significantly reduces its environmental footprint. Compared to the meat-heavy Western diet, the Mediterranean approach generates fewer greenhouse gas emissions, requires less water for food production, and utilizes land more efficiently. It also promotes sustainability by reducing the need for synthetic fertilizers, which benefits soil health and minimizes the environmental impact of fertilizer production. The Mediterranean diet's traditional reliance on locally sourced and diverse foods can support regional agriculture and promote biodiversity, contributing to a more resilient food system benefitting the environment.

Western diets typically feature a high proportion of meat, especially red meat. Livestock farming is a major contributor to climate change due to methane emissions, while also demanding significant land and water resources. They often rely heavily on processed and packaged foods, which involve energy-intensive manufacturing, packaging, and transportation processes. The Mediterranean diet, with its emphasis on fresh, seasonal, and minimally processed ingredients, reduces these environmental costs.

WHAT ABOUT OTHER HERITAGE DIETS?

The Mediterranean diet can be considered a *heritage diet* because it's based on long established food traditions that have a historical, cultural, and geographical context.

But there are similar traditional dietary patterns from other regions of the world that share the same characteristics, including low consumption of harmful saturated fats, trans fats, refined carbohydrates, and ultra-processed foods. These are plant-predominant diets high in unsaturated fats, fiber, whole grains, and legumes. There may also be specific foods, especially from colorful plants, that are rich in vitamins and minerals or bioactive compounds, which have anti-inflammatory effects and reduce oxidative stress.

There is every reason to have confidence that following any one of these diets will promote good management of cholesterol. The Mediterranean diet is the best defined and most studied heritage diet on the planet, and it may be just a matter of time before other traditional diets with origins in Africa, South America, or Asia reveal similar evidence to support their benefits to cholesterol management and overall health.

3

Assessing Risks

Learn how to calculate risk to prevent heart disease, stroke, and other complications.

Discover what primary prevention is and why it matters.

Understand how risk calculators work.

Identify how the risks affect you.

Chapter **7**

Calculating the Risk of Cholesterol

I n this chapter, we explain how your doctor will consider your lipid panel test and use tools to assess your risk of developing cardiovascular disease (CVD). The central person in any discussion about the management of your cholesterol and CVD risk should be *you*, so it's important for you to understand the basics about how these tools work. When you understand how the tools work, you'll be able to ask the right questions and feel that any decisions are truly shared by you and your doctor. That puts you in the driver's seat of any treatment plans, which is where you belong.

Understanding the Difference between Primary Prevention and Secondary Prevention

The medical approach to preventing CVD can be divided into two distinct situations: *primary prevention* and *secondary prevention*.

>> **Primary prevention:** Primary prevention focuses on stopping the disease before it starts. This applies to people who have never had heart disease, stroke, or other circulation-related problems but may have risk factors such as high cholesterol, high blood pressure, smoking, diabetes, or obesity. The goal is to keep the blood vessels healthy by making lifestyle changes, such as enjoying an excellent diet, exercising regularly, and avoiding smoking. In some cases, medications like statins, which lower cholesterol, may be recommended if a person's overall risk is high.

>> **Secondary prevention:** Secondary prevention is for people who already have CVD — meaning there is already evidence of atherosclerosis perhaps leading to symptoms of reduced blood flow to the heart, brain, limbs, or elsewhere. People in this category have a much higher risk of further complications, so treatment is more aggressive. Statins are almost always recommended, often at higher doses, and additional cholesterol- and blood pressure–lowering medications may be needed, as well as much greater attention to lifestyle modifications. The goal is to slow or even reverse the disease and reduce the risk of future heart attacks, strokes, or other serious events. We look at the treatment of CVD and secondary prevention in more detail in Chapter 11.

A key factor in deciding on treatment is whether a person has existing CVD. If someone has already had a heart attack, stroke, or other clear signs of blocked arteries, it's obvious they have CVD and need secondary prevention. Some people may have no symptoms but show early signs of atherosclerosis through tests like coronary artery calcium (CAC) scoring or ultrasound scans of their arteries. Tests may be carried out for people who are at high risk, or signs of CVD may be picked up during medical care for other reasons. These people are at high risk, even if they feel healthy. In some cases, doctors will treat them as if they have existing CVD, recommending cholesterol-lowering medication; in other cases, doctors may still treat them for primary prevention and those guidelines for treatment will be applied.

REMEMBER

There is no clear cutoff between someone who has some evidence of atherosclerosis, which is an almost inevitable consequence of aging, and someone whose degree of blood vessel disease may not yet be producing symptoms, but which is extensive enough to be defined as asymptomatic CVD. This is why doctors use a combination of risk calculators, medical history, and imaging tests to make the best decisions for each person.

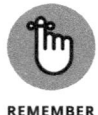

REMEMBER

When doctors use tools to assess the risk of developing CVD over a specific time frame, they are, by definition, using models developed specifically for the primary prevention of CVD, assuming there is no evidence of established disease.

Considering levels of risk in primary prevention

Everyone has a certain level of *circulating cholesterol* (cholesterol in the bloodstream), most of it in the form of a mixture of "bad" low-density lipoprotein (LDL) cholesterol and "good" high-density lipoprotein (HDL) cholesterol. When doctors talk about high cholesterol, they're usually referring to a high *cholesterol ratio*, which is the ratio of total cholesterol to HDL cholesterol.

Although high cholesterol is sometimes described as a disease and may even be referred to as *hypercholesterolemia*, in most contexts it can more accurately be viewed as a risk factor for developing diseases — like CVD — that are the consequence of poor blood flow to organs of the body that perform essential functions to maintain health and life.

In Chapter 2, we walk you through lipid panel results. There are ranges of figures for a cholesterol ratio that can be roughly defined as normal, borderline, or high, but in reality, the results are always somewhere on a spectrum and need to be judged in the context of other risk factors.

In recent years, algorithms have been introduced to compute some of the other measurable risk factors along with the cholesterol ratio, to produce a final calculation of approximate risk of developing CVD in the next ten years. We cover these tools later in this chapter.

Public health bodies and institutions have been able to gather all the scientific evidence about risk and the benefits of available treatments and have issued guidance to doctors with recommendations about when to intervene and how best to manage cholesterol.

Most guidelines suggest that medications, specifically statins, are recommended for individuals with a ten-year CVD risk of more than 20 percent, and should be considered, alongside lifestyle advice, in those with a risk above 7 percent to 10 percent, depending on the country you live in.

WARNING

The decisions of the expert guideline committees are based on the best available evidence, and committee members make a judgment about the thresholds for changing management advice. Although this judgment isn't arbitrary, it does come down to the views of the experts involved. Many guidelines take into account value for money of treatment options and also the costs of diseases to health systems. A significant proportion of medical studies are funded by the pharmaceutical industry, so it's essential that the quality of evidence be closely scrutinized and any conflicts of interest of the committee members, such as links to the pharmaceutical industry, be declared and managed appropriately.

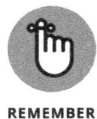

REMEMBER

Recommendations in guidelines are based on population statistics, but the way they're applied should be dependent on individual circumstances. For example, sometimes medications are contraindicated or may cause side effects, which means they aren't tolerated. In Chapter 8, we cover the importance of making decisions for you as an individual.

Treating for risk reduction

The discussion you may have with your doctor about whether to pursue treatment for your lipid panel results is informed by professional guidelines produced by public health bodies and organizations. In most cases, doctors follow the advice of the expert recommendations.

Guidelines from the National Institute for Health and Care Excellence (NICE) in the United Kingdom, the American Heart Association (AHA) and American College of Cardiology (ACC) in the United States, and the European Society of Cardiology (ESC) in Europe rely on multiple sources of high-quality scientific evidence to develop their recommendations. These organizations consider data from large-scale randomized controlled trials, long-term observational studies, risk prediction models, and safety analyses to ensure their guidelines reflect both the best available research and real-world clinical practice. They use this data to recommend when treatment should be considered. (See the nearby sidebar, "Where the Evidence Comes From," for more information.)

If treatment of your cholesterol level is recommended to reduce your risk of developing CVD, the first-line drug approach is with a medication called a *statin*. Statins are a class of medications used to lower cholesterol levels and reduce the risk of CVD. They work by inhibiting an enzyme in the liver that plays a key role in cholesterol production, helping to decrease levels of LDL cholesterol. By lowering LDL cholesterol, statins help prevent the buildup of fatty deposits in the arteries (see Chapter 2), which can lead to heart attacks and strokes. These drugs have become one of the most widely prescribed treatments for CVD prevention worldwide.

TECHNICAL STUFF

Statins work by inhibiting an enzyme called *HMG-CoA reductase,* which is crucial in the liver's cholesterol production process. By blocking this enzyme, statins reduce the amount of cholesterol produced, prompting the liver to remove more LDL cholesterol from the bloodstream. This leads to a significant reduction in LDL levels and, to a lesser extent, an increase in HDL cholesterol.

In addition to lowering cholesterol, statins have several other beneficial effects that help protect the heart and blood vessels. One of these effects is reducing inflammation in the walls of the arteries. Inflammation can cause damage to the blood vessels and is a key factor in the development of atherosclerosis.

Statins help reduce this inflammation, making the arteries less prone to damage and the buildup of plaque.

Another important effect of statins is that they help stabilize plaques that have already formed in the arteries. Plaques can sometimes rupture, leading to the formation of blood clots that can block blood flow, causing heart attacks or strokes. By stabilizing the plaque, statins make it less likely to break apart, reducing the risk of these dangerous events. This stabilization happens because statins help to make the plaques less inflamed and less likely to cause problems.

Statins also seem to reduce the oxidation of LDL cholesterol. Normally, when LDL cholesterol particles become oxidized, they can contribute to the buildup of plaque in the arteries. Oxidized LDL is more likely to trigger an inflammatory response, making it even more damaging to the blood vessels. Statins can reduce the oxidation of LDL, further helping to protect the arteries and reduce the risk of CVD.

Together, these effects — reducing inflammation, stabilizing plaques, and lowering LDL oxidation — add to the heart-protective benefits of statins, making them an effective treatment not just for lowering cholesterol but also for reducing the risk of heart attacks, strokes, and other heart-related issues. These combined effects make statins a powerful tool for preventing heart disease and stroke, although many health professionals are unaware of their beneficial effects on inflammation and oxidation and focus just on their ability to reduce the cholesterol numbers in the lipid panel result.

WARNING

Statins can have side effects. Some people are unable to take them for this and other reasons (see Chapter 11).

The decision about whether to use a statin, which is usually a decision for lifelong therapy, should be made by you and your doctor and needs to be based on the most up-to-date recommendations and guidelines, which use risk assessment tools (covered later in this chapter).

REMEMBER

The benefits of statins in reducing major vascular events are well-established, but a comprehensive understanding of their effects requires careful consideration of these limitations.

REMEMBER

Lifestyle changes to manage your cholesterol and reduce your risk of CVD should always be part of the discussion, and there should be a focus on shared decision-making. If your doctor uses a risk assessment tool, they can fill it in during a consultation and talk about the results and recommendations with you.

WHERE THE EVIDENCE COMES FROM

One of the most important sources of evidence has come from the Cholesterol Trialists' Collaboration (CTT), which is a research organization that collects and analyzes data from randomized controlled trials (RCTs) of cholesterol-lowering drugs, including statins. The CTT has conducted several assessments of these trials, which have provided strong evidence for the benefits of statins in primary prevention of CVD. In its 2012 publication, the CTT analyzed data from 27 RCTs involving more than 170,000 participants. It found that statin therapy reduced the risk of major coronary events (such as heart attack and stroke) by about 25 percent for every 38.7 mg/dL (1.0 mmol/L) reduction in LDL cholesterol. This benefit was seen across a wide range of baseline LDL cholesterol levels and in people with different levels of CVD risk. Based on this evidence, NICE, the ESC, and the AHA/ACC now recommend considering statin therapy for primary prevention of CVD in people with a ten-year risk of 7.5 percent to 10 percent or higher.

The CTT's work, though widely respected, is not without its critics. One key area of concern revolves around data access. Although the CTT collaborates with trial investigators, it doesn't always have access to the complete, individual, patient-level data from every trial included in its meta-analyses. This lack of full transparency raises questions about independent verification and the potential for bias, especially given that many of the original trials are funded by pharmaceutical companies. Critics also point to the CTT's primary focus on major vascular events, like heart attacks and strokes. Although these events are undeniably important, some argue that this focus may downplay other potential adverse effects of statins, such as muscle problems or the development of diabetes.

The CTT combines results from many studies on statins. However, these studies aren't all identical. They can differ in how they're designed. For example, each study may include or exclude different types of patients, use slightly different treatment plans, or measure health outcomes in different ways. These variations across studies make it more difficult to draw broad conclusions that apply to everyone. It's like trying to understand the effects of a medicine when it has been tested in slightly different ways on different groups of people — the overall picture is more complex.

Another issue is the possibility of "publication bias." Studies that show statins work well are more likely to get published in medical journals than studies that show little or no benefit. This can create a misleading impression that statins are more effective than they actually are, because the less positive results are hidden. Although the CTT tries to find all the studies, published or not, this bias can still be a problem.

Finally, although the CTT itself doesn't receive money from drug companies, many of the original studies it uses were funded by the companies that make statins. This raises concerns about potential conflicts of interest. Even if unintentional, the drug companies' funding could influence how the studies were designed, how the data were analyzed, and how the results were reported. It's important to remember these points when considering the evidence for statins.

Making Sense of Risk Assessment Tools

Doctors and public health experts use risk assessment tools and algorithms to predict a person's chance of developing serious health problems before they happen. These tools are based on large studies that track thousands, sometimes millions, of people over time. By analyzing patterns in health, lifestyle, and medical conditions, researchers can create formulas that estimate a person's future risk of diseases like heart attacks, strokes, or diabetes. The goal is to identify those who would benefit most from early treatment or lifestyle changes, helping to prevent illness rather than just treating it after it occurs.

These risk calculators combine different pieces of personal health information — such as age, cholesterol level, blood pressure, smoking habits, and medical history — to produce a percentage score that represents the likelihood of developing a disease over a set period, usually ten years. This approach allows doctors to make more informed decisions about who needs medication, who may be able to manage their risk through lifestyle changes, and who is already at low risk. Tools like QRISK and Atherosclerotic Cardiovascular Disease (ASCVD) scoring systems are widely used in routine healthcare to guide these decisions, ensuring that prevention strategies are based on solid scientific evidence rather than guesswork.

The tools have developed in recent years and can incorporate, quantify, and weigh up more than just the well-known risk factors like your cholesterol ratio, age, blood pressure, smoking status, a diagnosis of diabetes, and a family history of CVD. A high body mass index (BMI), the presence of certain diseases or medications associated with CVD, or the systemic inflammation that can increase the likelihood of developing CVD have been added to the list.

WARNING

You may look at a risk assessment tool and realize that it doesn't include your excellent (or poor) dietary habits or how frequently you exercise. These aspects of lifestyle are difficult to measure, but they have a profound influence on your risk of developing CVD. It may also occur to you that most algorithms don't include measurements of oxidized LDL cholesterol and inflammation. These represent very important gaps in the assessment of your risk. Chapter 8 is all about how to assess your *individual* risk.

The ASCVD Risk Estimator

The ASCVD Risk Estimator (`https://tools.acc.org/ascvd-risk-estimator-plus`) is a widely used tool in the United States for estimating a person's risk of developing heart disease or having a stroke over the next ten years. It was developed by the ACC and the AHA using data from large population studies. This calculator helps doctors assess whether someone would benefit from cholesterol-lowering medication, such as statins, or other preventive measures. It takes into account factors such as cholesterol levels, blood pressure, age, smoking status, diabetes, and lifestyle habits. Unlike some other risk calculators, ASCVD also includes race as a factor, because research has shown that cardiovascular risk can differ among different ethnic groups.

The ACC and AHA generally recommend that individuals with a ten-year risk of 7.5 percent or higher consider treatment with statin medications, though this decision is often adjusted based on personal health history and preferences.

The QRISK Risk Calculator

In England, the QRISK Risk Calculator (`https://qrisk.org`) serves a similar purpose in predicting CVD risk. Developed by medical researchers using extensive data from UK patients, QRISK is regularly updated to improve accuracy and ensure that it reflects changes in population health. The NICE recommends QRISK as a standard tool for guiding decisions about cholesterol management and heart disease prevention. Like ASCVD, QRISK considers cholesterol levels, blood pressure, smoking, diabetes, and other health factors, but it also includes additional elements such as BMI and certain long-term conditions like chronic kidney disease. Doctors in the UK typically consider a QRISK score of 10 percent or higher as a threshold for recommending preventive treatment, including lifestyle changes and possibly statins to lower cholesterol. QRISK is updated periodically when more evidence becomes available.

The questions asked in QRISK are ideally completed by you and your doctor using the online tool. Each answer is associated with a particular risk profile and is weighed accordingly. When you click the Calculate Risk button, you're shown a final figure that represents your risk of developing CVD in the next ten years.

Other algorithms

Although QRISK and ASCVD are prominent, several others are used globally. Here are a few notable examples:

>> **Systematic Coronary Risk Evaluation 2 (SCORE2):** Developed by the European Society of Cardiology, SCORE2 is a widely used risk prediction model in Europe. It estimates the ten-year risk of fatal and nonfatal cardiovascular events in individuals aged 40 to 69 years. In common with other tools, it considers factors like age, sex, smoking status, blood pressure, and cholesterol levels. SCORE2 has been updated and recalibrated to improve its accuracy and applicability across different European regions.

>> **Framingham Risk Score:** This is one of the oldest and most widely used risk assessment tools globally. It was developed based on data from the Framingham Heart Study and estimates the ten-year risk of coronary heart disease. It takes into account age, sex, total cholesterol, HDL cholesterol, blood pressure, smoking status, and diabetes. Although it has been around for a while, it's still a valuable tool, especially in primary-care settings.

>> **Reynolds Risk Score:** This risk score adds high-sensitivity C-reactive protein (hs-CRP) to traditional risk factors. hs-CRP is a marker of inflammation, and its inclusion can improve risk prediction, particularly in women. It also considers family history of heart disease, which can be an important risk factor.

>> **Pooled Cohort Equations:** Developed by the AHA and the ACC, these equations are used in the United States to estimate the ten-year risk of atherosclerotic CVD. They consider a wide range of factors, including age, sex, race, blood pressure, cholesterol level, diabetes, smoking status, and use of certain medications.

>> **InterHeart Risk Score:** This risk score was developed based on data from the InterHeart study, a large international study that examined risk factors for heart attack. It estimates the ten-year risk of heart attack and considers factors like age, sex, smoking status, blood pressure, cholesterol level, diabetes, obesity, and psychosocial factors.

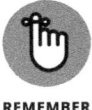

REMEMBER

Whichever model is used, they generally use similar data and risk factors and share predictive strengths and weaknesses, which may be significant for you as an individual (see Chapter 8). Understanding your *individual* risk for cholesterol-related complications is key to maintaining optimal health.

Chapter **8**

Understanding Your Individual Risk

The majority of people in the United States and Europe will have their cholesterol measured in a lipid panel test at some point in their lives, and for many, this will be a regular event. After the test, you should have a conversation with your doctor about what the results mean for you.

If you've been diagnosed with cardiovascular disease (CVD), have a genetic condition called familial hypercholesterolemia (FH), or have other medical conditions that put you at a very high risk of CVD, the case for treatment to lower your cholesterol is compelling. Treatment for *secondary prevention* (aimed at preventing further cardiovascular events in individuals already diagnosed with CVD) dramatically reduces the risk of further complications of CVD. You'll almost certainly be advised to take statins or other medications (see Chapter 11).

If you've had the test done as a screening or as part of a health check, with the assumption that you don't have existing CVD, a decision about the result is usually made using a primary prevention risk assessment tool, like the ones we cover in this chapter.

In this chapter, you get to know the risk tools your doctor will use, appreciate their limitations, and find the right questions to ask your doctor to come to a shared decision about how best to manage your cholesterol.

Interpreting the Risks

If your doctor has asked you to make an appointment to discuss your lipid panel test results, they'll almost certainly ask you other questions about your general health, other risk factors, and lifestyle. Those questions will include your age, gender, ethnicity, smoking history, and a series of questions about other medical conditions like diabetes. Your doctor may also measure your height, weight, and blood pressure. (Turn to Chapter 7 for the complete list.) Your doctor will then plug this information into one of the recommended risk tool assessments (for example, QRISK or ASCVD) and present you with some information to consider together.

Knowing what a risk score means for you

To fully understand what a risk score means for you, you need to know the difference between *absolute risk* and *relative risk.* Relative risk reduction shows how much an intervention or treatment reduces risk compared to the original risk, while absolute risk reduction shows the actual difference in risk percentages caused by the intervention or treatment.

Imagine 100 people have a certain level of heart disease risk. Let's say 5 of them are expected to have a heart attack over the next ten years. That's a 5 percent risk. Now, imagine they all take a statin. If the statin reduces the risk by 20 percent, the number of people expected to have a heart attack would drop to 4 people. Relative risk reduction looks at the percentage change. In this case, the risk went down by one out of five people, which is a 20 percent reduction. This sounds impressive!

Absolute risk reduction, on the other hand, looks at the *actual* difference in risk. Here, the risk went down by 1 percentage point (from 5 percent to 4 percent). This may seem less dramatic than the relative reduction.

REMEMBER

Both numbers are important, but they tell different stories. The relative risk reduction can make a treatment seem very effective, especially when the initial risk is low. But the absolute risk reduction gives you a clearer picture of the actual impact on your chances of having a heart attack. For example, if your initial risk is very low (say 1 percent), a 50 percent relative risk reduction may only translate to a 0.5 percent absolute risk reduction. This may not be a big enough change to be meaningful for you.

TIP

It's important to discuss both absolute and relative risk reduction with your doctor. They can help you understand the numbers in the context of your own health and make informed decisions about your treatment.

Some of the tools we mention provide an absolute risk and a relative risk — comparing your risk with how an average, healthy individual may measure up. QRISK provides a "heart age," which compares the model's conclusions with a healthy average and calculates whether your "heart age" is older or younger than your actual age.

Here's an example, for a 62-year-old, nonsmoking male with a systolic (upper measurement) blood pressure of 130, a body mass index (BMI) in the normal range (though close to the upper limit) and a total cholesterol–to–high-density lipoprotein (HDL) cholesterol ratio at the upper limit of desirable at 5.0:

10-year QRISK score: 12 percent

The score of a healthy person with the same age, sex, and ethnicity*:
9.7 percent

Relative risk:** 1.2 percent

QRISK Healthy Heart Age*:** 66

* This is the score of a healthy person the same age, sex, and ethnic group, with no adverse clinical indicators and a cholesterol ratio of 4.0, a stable systolic blood pressure of 125, and BMI of 25.

** Relative risk is an individual's risk divided by a healthy person's risk.

*** The QRISK Healthy Heart Age is the age at which a healthy person of the same sex and ethnicity has the same ten-year QRISK score.

If this 62-year-old person instead had a cholesterol, BMI, and blood pressure that was midrange for their age, their risk of developing CVD over ten years would be 9.7 percent; their heart age would, at 62, be the same as their actual age; and their relative risk would be exactly 1, rather than 1.2. Each 0.1 increment above 1.0 represents a 10 percent increase in relative risk, so being at the upper limits of cholesterol, BMI, and blood pressure places them at a 20 percent relative increased risk.

REMEMBER

This all may seem a little scary, but it's important to put this in context by realizing that these tools don't tell the whole story of you, your life, and your risk. Put another way, you can keep your risks of CVD low and enjoy a lifestyle that keeps you fit and healthy.

Recognizing the limitations of risk tools

CVD risk assessment tools, which use cholesterol levels and other criteria to create a primary prevention risk profile, have limitations. The algorithms often focus on a select number of traditional risk factors, neglecting a broader spectrum of lifestyle and emerging biomarkers that significantly influence CVD risk. For instance, factors like exercise levels, dietary habits, the composition of the gut microbiome, and chronic stress are generally left out of the commonly used assessments. These omissions can lead to an incomplete picture of an individual's true risk, potentially underestimating or overestimating their likelihood of developing CVD. A person with a healthy diet and active lifestyle may have a lower actual risk than their score suggests, while someone with poor lifestyle habits may be at greater risk than the tool indicates.

Although a healthier lifestyle may make a difference to the measured cholesterol levels, blood pressure, and BMI, the actual benefits will never be fully assessed by a tool that doesn't attach any importance to lifestyle.

REMEMBER

Regular exercise can reduce CVD risk by 20 percent to 30 percent independently of other factors. The Mediterranean diet can lower risk by 25 percent to 30 percent. These effects are not marginal — they have an impact greater than most of the criteria included in the calculations and greater than the effects of statins, which are often recommended after using these tools.

TIP

Most risk tools don't include diet and exercise in part because they're difficult to measure. There is no laboratory test that can measure diet and exercise. The *medical model of care* — the traditional approach to healthcare that focuses primarily on diagnosing and treating physical illnesses — has a history of not paying enough attention to *lifestyle medicine,* which uses evidence-based lifestyle changes to prevent, treat, and reverse chronic diseases. When it comes to risk tools, it's important to remember the words attributed to William Bruce Cameron, an expert on measurement systems: "Not everything that can be counted counts, and not everything that counts can be counted."

WARNING

Doctors shouldn't ignore the effects of the factors excluded from the risk assessment calculators. It's possible for two people with the same characteristics, measured numbers, and reported risk to have very different lifestyles — one may exercise regularly and enjoy a healthy Mediterranean diet rich in antioxidant and anti-inflammatory nutrients and bioactive compounds, and the other may have a very poor diet and sedentary lifestyle. Evidence is clear that these two individuals have very different risks of developing CVD, but it may not be adequately captured by the risk tools.

Another limitation stems from the inclusion of unmodifiable risk factors like age, sex, and family history. These factors are undeniably associated with CVD risk, but they can't be altered through lifestyle changes or interventions. Including them in risk calculations can create a sense of inevitability, particularly for older people. As we age, the inherent probability of experiencing a cardiovascular event or death increases, leading to naturally higher risk scores in these age groups. This can sometimes obscure the potential benefits of lifestyle modifications or medical interventions, even if they significantly reduce relative risk. It's crucial to remember that even with unmodifiable risk factors, lifestyle changes can still substantially impact overall cardiovascular health. As age increases, the number of people whose doctors recommend treatment rises dramatically. Of all the criteria in risk tools, age is the most influential on risk, the most likely to result in medication, and the least able to be influenced or changed!

Another blunt assessment criterion is the question of a family history of early heart disease. This makes no distinction between a family member living a healthy life but developing early CVD due to genetic influences and one who may have smoked 40 cigarettes a day, had diabetes, and succumbed to CVD because of lifestyle factors. The first scenario may suggest a link with further generations, whereas the second would be much less likely to affect a person who had a different lifestyle.

Some of the criteria used in CVD risk assessment tools can be imprecise and subject to misinterpretation. BMI, for example, is a widely used metric, but it fails to distinguish between muscle mass and fat. A highly muscular individual may be classified as overweight or obese based on BMI alone, despite having a low percentage of body fat and a healthy metabolic profile. Population studies don't make distinctions between people with an "unhealthy" or "healthy" high BMI. Similarly, blood pressure measurements taken in a clinical setting can be influenced by the "white coat effect," where anxiety about the appointment temporarily elevates blood pressure. A single reading may not accurately reflect an individual's typical blood pressure throughout the day, potentially leading to an inaccurate risk assessment.

Finally, traditional CVD risk assessments often overlook more sensitive and specific biomarkers that provide a deeper understanding of cardiovascular health. Oxidized low-density lipoprotein (LDL) cholesterol and markers of inflammation, such as high-sensitivity C-reactive protein (hs-CRP), are increasingly recognized as important contributors to atherosclerosis and plaque development. These markers can provide valuable insights into an individual's risk beyond what traditional risk factors reveal. For example, someone with normal cholesterol levels but elevated hs-CRP may be at increased risk of plaque formation and future cardiovascular events. The absence of these more nuanced biomarkers in standard risk assessment tools can limit their predictive accuracy and potentially miss individuals who are at higher risk despite seemingly normal traditional markers.

Beyond these established limitations, several other factors contribute to the complexity of CVD risk assessment. Some tools try to incorporate aspects of socioeconomic status, mental health, and even race and ethnicity, but these are often simplified and may not fully capture the nuanced interplay of these factors with individual risk. Socioeconomic factors, such as access to healthy food and safe exercise environments, can significantly influence CVD risk independently of traditional risk factors. Similarly, mental health conditions like depression and anxiety are strongly associated with increased risk, yet are rarely addressed comprehensively in risk assessments. Even when race and ethnicity are included, they often fail to account for the complex interaction of genetics, culture, and socioeconomic disparities that contribute to varying risk profiles across populations.

The impact of medications on CVD risk, both positive and negative, is often not fully considered either, particularly in older adults who may be taking multiple medications.

It's also important to recognize that risk assessment tools typically provide a static snapshot of risk at a specific point in time and don't dynamically reflect changes in lifestyle or the initiation of medical interventions. This can limit their value in tracking the effectiveness of risk-reduction strategies.

Ultimately, it's crucial to acknowledge that these tools provide a probability, not a certainty, and their results should be interpreted cautiously in the context of a comprehensive clinical, individual evaluation. They're valuable tools for informing, but not dictating, clinical decisions.

REMEMBER

If you follow a Mediterranean diet and exercise regularly, your "true" CVD risk is likely lower than the standard risk assessment tools would predict. Conversely, someone who scores "low risk" on these tools but has a poor diet and sedentary lifestyle may have a higher actual risk than estimated.

Working with Your Doctor to Treat (or Not Treat) Your Cholesterol

When it comes to treatment of cholesterol to lower the risk of CVD, most doctors recommend that patients take a statin (see Chapter 11). Unfortunately, this approach taken by many physicians misses the opportunity to discuss lifestyle measures to reduce cholesterol, to lower its oxidation and inflammation, and to independently and additionally reduce the risk of CVD. This book is intended to fill that gap and to support you in your discussions with your doctor about cholesterol management and treatment.

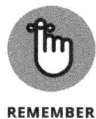

REMEMBER

Making positive lifestyle changes is a great idea whatever your cholesterol and CVD risk calculation. It may be all you need, especially if your ten-year CVD risk is below 10 percent. It may be an alternative to statins for those with intermediate risk, and it certainly goes hand in hand with medication if it's necessary for higher risk levels.

There's no doubt that health systems that screen people for cholesterol, assess ten-year CVD risk, and recommend statin treatment for anyone with a risk greater than 7.5 percent to 10 percent dramatically drive up statin use. Most people over the age of 60, especially men, with typical values put into the algorithms, will find themselves with a risk calculation of more than 7.5 percent or 10 percent, which are the thresholds in the United States and Europe, respectively, above which statins are frequently prescribed.

However, with the limitations of the tools, as well as the pros and cons of taking statins, each decision to decline, defer, initiate, or stop such treatment must be weighed individually.

REMEMBER

Making lifestyle changes is always important, whether you're going to take medications or not. It's always the first place to start, with medications added only if your risk of CVD is high and you and your doctor decide that's best. When you're taking medications, it's crucial that you continue to make healthy decisions because they're beneficial in their own right.

Knowing when to start or stop statins

There are no absolute right or wrong answers about using statins to treat cholesterol. There is no doubt that treatment can be very effective for people at high risk with existing CVD or significant risk factors, but the advantages of taking statins may be very marginal or nonexistent at lower risk levels. The discussion with your doctor should encompass these subtleties.

TIP

Statin benefit is proportional to absolute risk, so if your risk is high, you'll get a greater benefit. If your risk is low — and especially if your true risk is lower than estimated — you may not gain meaningful benefit from taking a statin.

REMEMBER

Although statins are considered very safe in general use, they do have the potential for side effects. If you experience side effects from statins, they may be mild. Sometimes, however, one or more side effects may be enough to merit changing or stopping it. Very rarely, side effects may be severe and even life threatening. There are some circumstances where statins are contraindicated, and others where they can interfere with other medications. We explore all these subjects in more depth in Chapter 11.

THE RISKS OF OVERTREATMENT

Some doctors are concerned about the "medicalization" of vast swathes of populations for the good of population health, with less clear benefits to individuals. Experts have called for much more open discussions between doctors and patients about when to start or stop medications for cholesterol. Professor David Haslam, the greatly respected former chief of the National Institute for Health and Care Excellence (NICE) which provides evidence-based guidance and recommendations to improve health and social care in England, has written on this subject in his book *Side Effects: How Our Healthcare Lost Its Way and How We Fix It* (published by Atlantic Books).

According to Professor Haslam, many discussions between doctors and patients are not as individually tailored and as thorough as they should be, especially given that the vast majority of people taking statins will not receive any benefit at all. Only a few of those taking the medication will, because of them, avoid a heart attack or stroke. Here's the example he gives: Let's say a group of 100 individuals is at 10 percent risk of developing CVD in ten years if none of them received statin treatment — that means 10 people would develop CVD. If all of them receive a statin, however, 4 would be saved from having a stroke or heart attack, 6 would go on to develop CVD anyway despite treatment, and 90 would be free of CVD, irrespective of treatment so they would've taken medication for ten years for no purpose.

The trouble is, it's not possible to identify in advance which group any individual may be in. How you look at the advantages and disadvantages depends on whether you're one of the four for whom there is a beneficial effect of treatment or one of the 90 who don't benefit — but it's impossible to know in advance.

WARNING

Though generally safe and effective, there are people for whom the benefits of statins for *primary prevention* (preventing the first occurrence of CVD in individuals at risk) may not outweigh the potential risks or burdens:

>> **Patients with very low baseline risk:** If someone has a very low ten-year risk of CVD, the absolute benefit from statin therapy may be small. In someone at very low risk, the small potential benefit may not outweigh the small but real risk of side effects, especially if they're otherwise healthy. Patients with a low or intermediate risk who adhere to a Mediterranean diet, engage in regular vigorous exercise, and have excellent control of other modifiable risk factors not measured by risk tools may have a lower *actual* risk than their calculated score suggests.

>> **People who experience muscle aches or other side effects when taking statins, making it difficult or impossible for them to continue treatment:** Although there are strategies for managing statin intolerance (such as trying

different statins or doses), in some cases the side effects may be severe enough that the risks of continuing statin therapy outweigh the potential benefits for primary prevention. In these situations, alternative approaches to risk reduction, such as lifestyle changes and other medications if appropriate, are even more important.

» **People with certain medical conditions that may increase the risk of side effects or make it more challenging to manage statin therapy:** For example, patients with liver or kidney disease may require closer monitoring or dose adjustments, and the presence of these conditions could tip the risk–benefit balance, particularly for primary prevention. Similarly, certain medications can interact with statins, increasing the risk of side effects. A careful review of the patient's medical history and current medications is essential before starting statin therapy.

» **People who have significant anxiety about the potential side effects of statins, even if their actual risk is low:** This anxiety can negatively impact quality of life, as well as affect compliance with treatment. In these situations, a thorough discussion about the risks and benefits of statin therapy, as well as strategies for managing side effects, is crucial. If the patient's anxiety is substantial, it may be reasonable to explore alternative approaches to risk reduction and make a shared decision to manage risk without medications.

» **People who are very elderly:** As people age, their risk of cardiovascular events naturally increases, but so does their risk of experiencing side effects from medications. In very old individuals, particularly those with multiple other health conditions or limited life expectancy, the benefits of statins in preventing a cardiovascular event many years down the line may be less impactful than the potential for muscle aches, liver problems, or interactions with other medications. The focus in this population often shifts toward maintaining quality of life and managing existing conditions rather than aggressively preventing future events that may not occur within their remaining lifespan. The decision to use a statin in this group should be made carefully on an individual basis, considering their overall health, life expectancy, and personal preferences.

» **People with terminal illnesses:** When someone has a limited life expectancy due to a terminal illness, the long-term benefits of statin therapy become less relevant. The focus of care in these situations is typically on comfort and *palliative care* (holistic support to improve quality of life for patients and their families facing life-limiting illnesses) instead of preventing future cardiovascular events. Adding a medication like a statin, which may not provide any immediate benefit and could potentially cause side effects, may not be the most appropriate approach. In these circumstances, it's important to prioritize the patient's comfort and well-being over long-term prevention strategies.

If a person takes medications like statins over many years, their circumstances can change as time goes on. It's important for doctors to regularly discuss with patients whether they're still benefiting from their medications and if their needs have evolved.

Talking with your doctor about treatment

When you talk with your doctor about your cholesterol and risk, it's important to feel that your views are being taken onto account and that you come away with answers to your questions. This may include your doctor telling you that it's not possible to give an answer!

In some cultures it's common for the doctor-patient relationship to be paternalistic, with the doctor making decisions with little discussion because "doctor knows best." In other countries, the patient may be more of a "consumer"; they may have seen TV advertisements encouraging them to take medication, assuming their insurance will pay for it. Some public health systems are under such pressure that important lifelong management decisions are made in a few minutes after a quick phone conversation.

It's really important that you feel empowered to ask questions and that you truly share in the decision-making process with your doctor.

Whether you decide to take a statin will depend on your attitude to risk, your values, and your view of committing to taking medication regularly. Of course, your doctor should tell you if they feel you're exposing yourself to unnecessarily high risks of illness, but you should be able to make up your own mind with their support. If your risk is low or only slightly raised, it's very acceptable to say no to medication.

Guidelines are exactly that — guidelines. They're based on population health. The final choice is a personal one.

The CVD risk reduction that comes with taking a statin for primary prevention is a statistical estimate, and like the risk assessment tools themselves, it's based on population data. The possible gains from taking a statin that your doctor quotes may not precisely apply to you as an individual because there are limitations of the algorithms. Not everyone will be helped by taking a statin for primary prevention of CVD, but some people will be.

There are two specific questions that can help you understand the merits of taking a statin, especially for people whose ten-year risk of developing CVD is calculated to be between 7.5 percent and 20 percent, where it's recommended to consider treatment: What are the "numbers needed to treat" and what is the reduction in absolute risk.

>> **What is the number needed to treat (NNT)?** The NNT refers to the number of people who need to take a statin for a certain period (for example, five years) to prevent one cardiovascular event (for example, a heart attack or stroke). For primary prevention of CVD, NNT varies based on individual risk factors, but it's often around 50 to 100 in low-risk populations.

There is also a concept of the number needed to harm (NNH), which represents how many people need to take a statin before one person experiences a significant adverse effect, such as muscle pain or diabetes. NNH is typically higher than NNT, often in the range of 100 to 200, meaning side effects are less frequent than the benefits in appropriately selected patients.

Balancing NNT and NNH helps determine whether statins are worthwhile for an individual without existing CVD.

>> **What is the reduction in absolute risk?** One of the common misperceptions about treatment with statins is that they'll provide complete protection from CVD. Just because a person is taking statins doesn't mean they won't develop CVD — it just reduces the risk.

For any starting risk, it's possible to calculate an approximate benefit for an average person who takes and tolerates a statin medication, using population data to calculate expected reductions in LDL cholesterol and CVD.

Let's take an individual with a 13 percent ten-year cardiovascular risk according to the QRISK tool. Initiating statin therapy can reduce the average risk of populations with a 13 percent starting risk. Statins are known to lower LDL cholesterol by approximately 30 percent, and for every 1 mmol/L (approximately 38.7 mg/dL) reduction in LDL, the risk of cardiovascular events decreases by about 22 percent. Therefore, the original 13 percent risk may decrease by about 2.86 percent (which is 22 percent of 13 percent), resulting in a new estimated ten-year risk of approximately 10.14 percent. That may seem a lot or it may seem marginal, depending on your viewpoint.

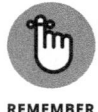

REMEMBER

This risk doesn't take into account oxidation of LDL, diet, and lifestyle which aren't assessed by the tool and which may make a difference to an individual's response to a statin.

Discuss these questions with your doctor and ask them to calculate the benefits for you as an individual. We explore potential side effects of taking statins or other cholesterol-lowering medication in Chapter 11.

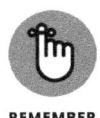

REMEMBER

Despite trying to be objective, the view your doctor has of your risk will inevitably be influenced by their attitude to risk.

MORE ACCURATE RISK TOOLS OF THE FUTURE

In the future, more information may be available and more detailed tests may be more widely accessible to make a more personalized and accurate judgment about whether to treat cholesterol with statins. There will surely be a role for artificial intelligence (AI) as well.

Risk assessment may include more questions about the frequency and types of exercise you engage in and your dietary pattern to indicate effects on oxidative stress and inflammation. For example, it would be possible for a "Mediterranean diet score" to be incorporated into algorithms to reflect the powerful positive effects on risk reduction.

One promising tool is the coronary artery calcium (CAC) scan. This low-dose CT scan measures the buildup of calcium in your heart's arteries, giving a direct look at plaque accrual instead of just estimating risk. A score of zero on this scan often means a very low risk, even if traditional risk calculators and tools suggest otherwise. Conversely, a high score can mean increased risk, even if other markers look good. CAC scans may be most useful people for people who have a small increased risk of CVD, which may be based more on crossing age thresholds than other factors. On the other hand, routine use of such scans would be expensive and, although radiation exposure is considered safe, it still needs to be taken into account.

Beyond the usual cholesterol numbers, advanced lipid testing will likely become more common. Instead of just LDL cholesterol, doctors may look at the number of LDL partcles and a protein called apolipoprotein B (ApoB), which are better predictors of heart disease. They may also check lipoprotein(a), or Lp(a) (pronounced L-P-little a), a genetically linked risk factor that isn't typically included in standard assessments. This means someone could have "normal" cholesterol levels but still be at risk due to these other factors. These advanced lipid tests can help identify people with a higher risk of heart disease despite having seemingly "normal" cholesterol levels, allowing for more targeted interventions.

Inflammation is another key player in heart disease (see Chapter 4). Some risk tools already include weighting for particular inflammatory conditions, but future assessments may take this further and include tests for hs-CRP, fibrinogen, and interleukin-6 (IL-6), all markers of inflammation. Endothelial function tests, which check how well your arteries are working based on the lining of the artery walls, could also become more common. Oxidized LDL, a marker of artery damage, may also be checked. These tests can help identify people more at risk even if their cholesterol level is fine.

Metabolic health, including how your body handles insulin and blood glucose, is also crucial. Tests for fasting insulin, measures of insulin resistance, and the ratio of triglycerides to HDL cholesterol could provide a more complete picture. This is important because someone with normal cholesterol but high triglycerides and insulin resistance could be at higher risk than traditional calculators suggest. These metabolic markers highlight the relationship between other health factors and their impact on heart disease risk.

Finally, technology is changing how we assess risk. Continuous glucose monitors (CGMs) can reveal hidden blood glucose spikes, while heart rate and variability tracking from smartwatches can provide insights into heart function — a low resting pulse and good variability indicate good cardiac health. Smart blood pressure monitors can capture fluctuations in blood pressure that single readings may miss. They're already being used by many patients to gain a more accurate insight into blood pressure.

By using more accurate assessments in the future, and increasing the accuracy of risk tools, a more personalized approach will empower individuals to take control of their heart health and make informed decisions about their lifestyle and treatment options.

IN THIS CHAPTER

» Understand the importance
of self-care

» Getting a good night's sleep

» Staying connected to family
and friends

Chapter **9**

Reducing Risk through Self-Care, Sleep, and Connection

The relationship between self-care, sleep, social connections, and cardio-vascular health, including effects on cholesterol, is an area of growing scientific interest. Pinpointing exact cause-and-effect relationships is complicated, but studies are increasingly highlighting the significant role of these lifestyle factors in cholesterol management.

REMEMBER

These elements are interconnected. For example, poor sleep can increase stress, which can negatively impact social connections and self-care practices. Studies provide strong evidence for the benefits of these lifestyle factors.

In this chapter, we explain how these aspects may relate to cholesterol, and show you how you can harness them as part of your cholesterol and cardiovascular health management plan.

Taking Time for Self-Care

Self-care is a bit of a buzzword these days, but in this case, it's worth all the hype. Self-care practices, including regular exercise and stress management, directly influence cardiovascular health. Exercise, for example, is well-documented for its ability to improve lipid profiles. Regular aerobic exercise significantly reduces low-density lipoprotein (LDL) cholesterol and increases high-density lipoprotein (HDL) cholesterol (see Chapter 10).

Stress-reduction techniques, such as mindfulness and meditation, have been shown to lower blood pressure and reduce the activity of the *sympathetic nervous system* (responsible for the "fight-or-flight" response), which is implicated in the development of cardiovascular disease (CVD). Studies published in the *Journal of Behavioral Medicine* have demonstrated that mindfulness-based interventions can lead to significant reductions in blood pressure and markers of inflammation.

TIP

If you're interested in meditation and you don't know where to begin, check out apps like Calm (www.calm.com) and Headspace (www.headspace.com). Meditation doesn't have to mean sitting in silence for hours like a Buddhist monk — it can be something you do for ten minutes in your car before heading into work.

WARNING

Several lifestyle factors are known to dramatically increase the risk of CVD:

>> **Smoking:** Smoking dramatically increases the risk of CVD. Quitting is hard, but you can do it with the right help. *Quitting Smoking & Vaping For Dummies,* by Charles H. Elliott and Laura L. Smith (published by John Wiley & Sons, Inc.), is a great place to start.

>> **Substance use disorder:** Substance use disorder encompasses everything from alcohol to opioids to marijuana and more. Sadly, in addition to being unhealthy for your mind and body, it increases your risk of CVD. If you're currently battling substance use disorder, talk with your doctor about treatment plans that may work for you.

>> **Poor diet:** Diet is directly tied to cholesterol and CVD. Parts 2 and 5 of this book are all about diet.

>> **Inactivity:** Staying active is another one of the main ways you can take care of yourself. (We cover the importance of activity for preventing CVD in Chapter 10.)

>> **Excess alcohol consumption:** Even if you don't consider yourself an alcoholic, you may be consuming too much alcohol, and that can increase the risk of CVD. The current guidelines are no more than two drinks per day for men and no more than one drink per day for women.

>> **Chronic stress:** Chronic stress isn't just occasionally feeling stressed out. It's a constant sense of being pressured or overwhelmed. Symptoms can include inability to focus, insomnia, and aches and pains.

Some harms are not easy to avoid, for example if you live in an area with poor air quality. Protective masks, with a minimum of N95 (USA standard) or FFP2 or 3 (European standard) can reduce exposure if you know that you are going to be exposed to pollutants in the environment.

TREATING ADDICTIONS

Addictions to processed and unhealthful foods, alcohol, cigarettes, and other substances are difficult to break. But if optimal health is your goal, it's worth exploring the options available to help heal and transform your addictions. Regardless of the type of addiction you may be facing, an underlying belief and pattern of habits is directly correlated to the harmful habit.

The keys to ending the vicious cycle of addiction and allowing your mind, body, and spirit to heal is to identify the original belief (lack of self-worth, the need for a coping mechanism, survival mentality, and so on) that fueled the addiction in the first place. When that idea is unlocked, with the help of the right person or program and a strong desire to change, you can transform the habits associated with the addiction.

Sometimes addictions are easy to sweep under the carpet because they aren't as dramatic as cases portrayed in movies and on the news. But the truth is, if an addiction to something or the inability to transform poor habits is impacting your life, it's worth working on. Mental health professionals, spiritual advisers, and health coaches are a wonderful first step if you don't know where to turn.

If you don't know where to turn, talk to your doctor to find reputable programs in your area (or those you can participate in online), as well as support groups that have proven track records of helping people overcome addiction to make way for a fulfilling lifestyle.

Getting Good-Quality Sleep

The importance of good-quality sleep for achieving a healthy cholesterol level and reducing the risk of CVD is becoming clearer. If you struggle to maintain a good sleep pattern, it's definitely worth trying techniques that can optimize your sleep.

TIP

The recommended sleep pattern for overall health varies by age, but for most adults, getting between seven to nine hours of sleep per night is ideal. Older adults (aged 65 and above) should aim for seven to eight hours per night.

In this section, we explain the importance of sleep and offer tips for how you can improve your sleep.

Seeing how sleep helps regulate cholesterol

Sleep plays a vital role in maintaining cardiovascular health, particularly in regulating cholesterol levels and controlling inflammation. Poor sleep quality and not getting enough sleep have been linked to changes in cholesterol metabolism. Sleep deprivation may reduce levels of HDL cholesterol while increasing levels of LDL cholesterol and triglycerides, both of which contribute to plaque buildup in the arteries. These effects can accelerate the development of atherosclerosis and increase the risk of heart disease and other CVDs.

One significant effect of poor sleep is an increased risk of high blood pressure, a major contributor to CVD. Both short sleep duration and insomnia have been associated with a higher likelihood of developing high blood pressure. High blood pressure can damage blood vessel walls and increase the likelihood of LDL accumulation, oxidation, and plaque formation.

Inadequate sleep can also lead to insulin resistance, a condition that disrupts the body's ability to regulate blood glucose and lipid levels. This disruption not only increases the risk of type 2 diabetes but also worsens lipid profiles by promoting higher triglyceride levels and lowering protective HDL cholesterol.

Hormonal regulation during sleep plays a key role in maintaining healthy cholesterol levels and overall cardiovascular function. During restful sleep, the body produces *melatonin,* a hormone that regulates the sleep-wake cycle and has antioxidant properties. Melatonin may help reduce oxidative stress and inflammation, both of which are linked to abnormal cholesterol levels and the progression of atherosclerosis.

In contrast, chronic sleep deprivation can lead to elevated levels of *cortisol,* the body's primary stress hormone. Excess cortisol increases the production of LDL cholesterol and triglycerides while contributing to insulin resistance and systemic inflammation. This hormonal imbalance not only heightens the risk of high blood pressure but also accelerates the formation of arterial plaque.

Improving your sleep

TIP

Maintaining a regular sleep schedule is essential for quality rest. Going to bed and waking up at the same time each day, including weekends, helps regulate the body's internal clock. Sleep should also be uninterrupted — your body should be allowed to progress through complete sleep cycles. Each cycle lasts approximately 90 minutes and includes light sleep, deep sleep, and rapid eye movement (REM) sleep. For most adults, completing four to six cycles per night is considered optimal. Aligning sleep times with the body's natural circadian rhythm by going to bed between 10 p.m. and midnight further enhances sleep quality and overall health.

TIP

Creating an environment conducive to rest is key. A cool, dark, and quiet bedroom promotes better sleep. The ideal room temperature is between 60°F and 67°F (15°C to 20°C).

REMEMBER

Limit your exposure to screens, such as phones and tablets, at least an hour before bedtime, because blue light can disrupt melatonin production. Additionally, avoiding stimulants like caffeine and alcohol in the hours leading up to sleep can prevent restlessness and fragmented sleep.

TIP

Here are some more ways to promote better sleep:

>> **Develop a nighttime ritual.** Setting aside time before you'd like to go to bed to help you unwind is beneficial. You can use this time to drink an herbal tea, write in a gratitude journal, take a warm bath, meditate, listen to soothing music or healing sounds (check out the many Hz, frequency, binaural beats, or Tibetan healing videos to support healing patterns on YouTube.) There are many types to choose from — use what feels best for you. You may also choose to practice yoga, sniff lavender essential oil, or keep a lavender plant in your room.

>> **Think about what you eat for dinner and when you eat it.** If you want to sleep well, eat a light meal for dinner. Choose foods that are rich in tryptophan, melatonin, magnesium, and omega-3 fatty acids because they may help you to relax. These foods include turkey, eggs, milk, cherries, cherry juice, walnuts, salmon, tuna, sardines, bananas, almonds, oatmeal, and rice.

>> **Discuss supplements with your healthcare professional.** Certain supplements such as magnesium (especially magnesium-L-threonate, or MgT),

5-hydroxytryptophan (5htp), melatonin, valerian, chamomile, and lemon balm may have properties that help to promote a better night's sleep, though the evidence is not clear cut. Talk about these options with your doctor, pharmacist, or nutritionist before trying them. Make sure they don't interact with any of your current medical conditions or medications and determine which would be best for you.

>> **Make sure that your hormones are balanced.** If you're going through a period of hormonal change (such as menopause) or extreme stress, you may want to ask your doctor to test your hormone levels. Inability to sleep properly is one of the symptoms of hormonal imbalances, so ruling this out and seeking advice is a good idea.

>> **Get moving.** Regular exercise impacts sleep by reducing stress and anxiety, regulating circadian rhythm, promoting relaxation, and helping you to fall asleep faster and experience longer periods of restful sleep. Try to stop exercising an hour or two before bed for optimal sleep. Exercising just before bed can raise your body temperature and make it harder to sleep. Keep in mind, though, that everyone is different. If the evening is the only time when you can exercise, or you feel that it helps you to sleep better or relax, go for it! Just be sure to avoid intense exertion before bed and allow sufficient cooldown time.

NAPPING

Sleep doesn't (and shouldn't) just occur at nighttime. Naps are very beneficial to health. They can help you to balance your hormones, avoid the afternoon slumps, increase alertness and productivity, improve overall sleep time in older adults, and reduce the risk of a cardiovascular event.

According to the National Sleep Foundation (NSF), naps can restore alertness, enhance performance, and reduce mistakes and accidents. A study at the National Aeronautics and Space Administration (NASA) on sleepy military pilots and astronauts found that a 40-minute nap improved performance by 34 percent and alertness by 100 percent.

Different kind of naps include

- **Recovery naps,** which help you make up for lost sleep at night.

- **Prophylactic naps,** which you take to prevent sleep loss. These are often used by night-shift workers before and during their shifts to prevent sleepiness on the job.

- **Appetitive naps** (think of a Mediterranean siesta), which are taken for the pleasure of doing so. They're known to improve mood and energy.

- **Fulfillment naps,** which are scheduled for children to ensure that they're getting enough sleep — but they're a good idea for adults as well.

- **Essential naps,** which are taken for those healing or fighting off illness.

Ideal nap times are believed to be between 10 and 20 minutes. Drinking a cup of coffee or tea before a nap can help you to not nap for more than 30 minutes, so the nap won't interact with your sleep in the evening.

Naps aren't always practical depending on your work setting. If you can't fit a nap in on workdays, try napping on your days off. If you can't sleep during the day, even a five- or ten-minute meditation can help you to relax and sleep better at night.

Keeping Connected

The importance of social connections in preventing CVD is an area of increasing research. The Mediterranean lifestyle is also well known for emphasizing the role of strong family and community relationships. Regions with exceptional longevity are also characterized by the presence of strong social bonds.

Understanding how connection helps

Research published in the *Proceedings of the National Academy of Sciences* demonstrated that individuals with well-developed social ties had lower levels of inflammatory markers, such as C-reactive protein, which are associated with increased cardiovascular risk. According to the "social buffering" hypothesis, social support helps mitigate the negative impact of stress and improves resilience. This may be explained by the fact that those with stronger social networks are more likely to engage in healthier behaviors, like regular exercise and healthy communal eating, and are less likely to experience chronic stress. Strong social relationships have even been associated with healthier lipid profiles, including lower levels of LDL cholesterol, which is known to contribute to the development of atherosclerosis. Emotional support from social networks may help regulate metabolic processes, reducing the production of harmful lipids and improving the body's ability to manage cholesterol levels.

A study in the *Journal of the American College of Cardiology* linked social isolation with a significantly increased risk of cardiovascular events, independent of other risk factors, with unfavorable changes in cholesterol metabolism. Individuals who are socially isolated are more likely to have higher levels of LDL cholesterol and triglycerides, both of which are associated with atherosclerosis. Social isolation also correlates with lower levels of HDL cholesterol. Chronic loneliness and stress can elevate circulating stress hormones like cortisol, which, over time, may impair lipid metabolism and increase LDL cholesterol. These physiological changes highlight how a lack of social connection can directly impact cholesterol regulation and increase the risk of atherosclerosis and CVD.

The mental health benefits of social ties may reinforce positive effect on cholesterol and cardiovascular protection. Strong social networks are associated with lower rates of anxiety and depression, conditions that can contribute to *dyslipidemia* (an imbalance of fat-carrying proteins in the bloodstream).

TECHNICAL STUFF

Biological processes linked to social relationships also play a significant role in cholesterol metabolism. Social support helps regulate the hypothalamic-pituitary-adrenal (HPA) axis, which controls the release of cortisol. Chronic stress resulting from social isolation can dysregulate this system, leading to increased cholesterol production and systemic inflammation. Reduced inflammation in those with strong social ties may improve lipid regulation and decrease the risk of plaque formation in the arteries.

Creating and maintaining connection

Physical activity and socializing and eating meals with others are foundations to the Mediterranean lifestyle, which is seen as the healthiest in the world. This is in stark contrast to a modern urban myth that depicts socialization and connection as nonessential activities that people engage in as entertainment. Modern societies encourage us to do things by ourselves and on our own. There's nothing wrong with that — in fact, at times it can be beneficial — but this type of mentality strengthens the misconception that connection isn't necessary or important to our health and happiness.

There is an old Italian adage, *Mente sana, corpo sano,* which means "Healthy mind, healthy body." Whether you're engaging in activities with others to improve your mood or your health is irrelevant, because they're both connected. Social connections promote healthy behaviors, strengthen the immune system, help you to feel more secure, and reduce stress, depression, and anxiety. Strong social bonds are the glue of Blue Zone areas of the world, where people live and perform well in their 90s and 100s.

A common denominator in the lifestyles of the world's healthiest communities is that people gather daily for communal meals. Residents on the Mediterranean island of Sardinia, for example, are ten times more likely to live past the age of 100 than people in the United States. In Sardinia, family-style eating is commonplace, and the practice is believed to contribute to the well-being of the residents. This is because there is something extremely satisfying and comforting about knowing that no matter what happens or how difficult life gets, at lunchtime you'll be surrounded with loved ones. This type of psychological security has a positive effect on health and happiness.

TIP

Fortunately, you don't have to move to a Mediterranean island to enjoy the type of psychological benefits that connection has to offer. Even if you live alone, you can create your own rituals and traditions to enjoy on a regular basis anywhere. Here are some ideas:

>> **Set up a communal meal ritual.** Whether it's breakfast, lunch, dinner, teatime, or a shared snack, find a time when you can meet with other people and enjoy something together. It doesn't have to be a romantic partner or family, it can be coworkers, neighbors, or friends. Studies show that you eat less, absorb more nutrients, and make better food choices when you eat with others as well.

>> **Go virtual.** One thing that the COVID-19 pandemic taught us was how to use technology to promote connection. Set up video calls with your friends and family from afar to enjoy meals together daily. Amy regularly "eats" with her friends and family in Italy and New York this way.

>> **Partner up.** Find a buddy for your favorite activities. Whether it's walking, gardening, playing sports, or participating in another hobby, having regular company for a pleasurable activity helps to promote connection.

>> **Join groups.** Meetup groups (www.meetup.com), classes, spiritual groups, and volunteering regularly are additional ways to meet like-minded people and enjoy activities together.

>> **Prioritize family and friends.** If you're fortunate enough to have family members and friends nearby, make a vow to engage with them more frequently and organize opportunities for connection — Sunday Suppers, weekly theme nights, and so on.

Scheduling time to connect with others is tough. Many people have barely enough time to do the "essentials" every day. When you decide that connection is key to your health, though, take time to seriously evaluate your schedule. Look for ways to swap out less healthful activities for those that promote connection time. Your overall heath will thank you for it.

Chapter **10**

Reducing Risk through Exercise and Stress Management

R egular exercise is one of the most effective ways to improve cholesterol levels and protect your blood vessels, ensuring a good blood supply to your heart, brain, and other essential organs. Diet plays a key role in cholesterol management, but physical activity has unique benefits that go beyond simply burning calories.

Chronic stress is increasingly recognized as a risk factor for cardiovascular disease (CVD), though its effects are more indirect than those of diet or exercise. Stress triggers a cascade of physiological responses that, over time, can contribute to unfavorable changes in cholesterol levels, promote inflammation, and affect the stability of arterial plaques. Short-term stress is a normal part of life, but persistent or poorly managed stress can place significant strain on the cardiovascular system, increasing the likelihood of heart disease and other cardiovascular conditions.

In this chapter, we explain the emerging evidence for the importance of these factors in your cholesterol management plan and offer some strategies you can use to enjoy beneficial exercise and reduce your stress level.

Enjoying Exercise

If you're trying to manage your cholesterol, it probably comes as no surprise that exercise should be a key component of your strategy. Exercise has numerous benefits for cholesterol in particular and health in general. In this section, we walk you through the specific benefits exercise offers and help you find a type of exercise you enjoy.

Recognizing the benefits of exercise

Research shows that exercise can help lower levels of low-density lipoprotein (LDL) cholesterol, often referred to as "bad" cholesterol, while increasing high-density lipoprotein (HDL) cholesterol, often referred to as "good" cholesterol. But the benefits don't stop there — exercise also helps reduce the risk of CVD by influencing inflammation, oxidation of LDL, and the stability of plaque in the arteries.

In the following sections, we offer more details on the benefits of exercise.

Seeing how exercise affects LDL and HDL

One of the key ways in which regular exercise improves cholesterol is by increasing the enzymes that help transport LDL from the blood to the liver, where it can be broken down and removed from the body. At the same time, exercise boosts HDL levels, which helps clear excess cholesterol from the bloodstream and transport it back to the liver for disposal. But it's not just about the amount of HDL — the *functionality* of HDL also improves with regular exercise. More efficient HDL particles are better at removing cholesterol from artery walls and preventing it from contributing to plaque buildup. This improved functionality makes exercise even more effective at reducing cardiovascular risk.

Reducing the oxidation of LDL cholesterol

Another way exercise protects against heart disease is by reducing the oxidation of LDL cholesterol, a key driver of plaque formation and instability.

Initially, physical activity increases oxidative stress because it raises the body's metabolic rate, leading to a temporary increase in the production of *free radicals* (unstable molecules that can damage cells, including LDL particles). However, over time, the body adapts to regular exercise by strengthening its antioxidant defenses, increasing the production of protective enzymes that neutralize free radicals and reduce overall oxidative stress. This long-term adaptation makes LDL less likely to oxidize, which is crucial because oxidized LDL triggers inflammation and attracts immune cells that contribute to plaque growth and instability. By strengthening the body's ability to manage oxidative stress, exercise creates a net protective effect against LDL oxidation and the damage it causes in the arteries.

Reducing inflammation

Inflammation is another major factor in CVD, and exercise has been shown to have powerful anti-inflammatory effects. Physical activity lowers levels of inflammatory markers such as C-reactive protein (CRP) and reduces the production of pro-inflammatory molecules that contribute to plaque formation and rupture. By keeping inflammation in check, exercise helps maintain healthier blood vessels and reduces the likelihood of dangerous blood clots forming inside narrowed arteries.

Perhaps one of the most overlooked benefits of exercise is its effect on plaque stability. Not all plaques are equally dangerous — some are more prone to rupture, which can trigger a heart attack. Exercise has been found to help stabilize plaques by promoting the development of a thicker, more protective fibrous cap around them, making them less likely to break apart. Additionally, exercise improves the function of the endothelium, the inner lining of blood vessels, helping to keep arteries flexible and responsive to changes in blood flow.

Other benefits of exercise

Exercising also

>> Builds muscle and helps maintain strong bones.

>> Improves sleep quality (see Chapter 9).

>> Reduces stress and anxiety.

>> Offers mood-boosting effects by releasing chemicals in the brain that promote happiness.

>> Helps manage symptoms of mental health conditions.

>> Improves memory, attention, and problem-solving skills.

>> Improves body image and self-confidence.

>> Stimulates digestion, promotes regular bowel movements, and prevents constipation.

>> Improves overall stamina, energy level, and endurance.

>> Promotes blood flow to the skin, which improves its appearance.

>> Can lead to a longer and healthier life expectancy.

REMEMBER

Consult with your healthcare professional before beginning a new exercise program.

Choosing the exercise that's right for you

TIP

Current guidelines issued by the World Health Organization (WHO) and the American Heart Association (AHA) recommend at least 150 minutes of moderate-intensity aerobic exercise or 75 minutes of vigorous exercise per week. Incorporating resistance training into your fitness regimen a couple of times a week can also be beneficial. Studies have indicated that although aerobic exercise has a more pronounced effect, resistance training contributes to improvements in lipid profiles, particularly when combined with aerobic activities.

When you're deciding which type of exercise to do, the most important thing is to find something you *enjoy*. All types of hobbies and daily activities have health benefits. Dancing, gardening, running, cooking, baking, even household chores can add up to help you achieve your physical activity goals. Whether you enjoy jogging, shooting hoops, biking, going to the gym, power walking, or playing tennis, engaging in the activity regularly can be effective in lowering your heart rate, improving your mood, and reducing stress.

One of the most unique aspects of the Mediterranean lifestyle is that most people living there don't set aside time to do formal exercise. That's because their lifestyles — which include gardening, household maintenance, preparing food from scratch, and lots of walking — provides them with the movement they need to stay happy and healthy. Those who live in urban areas and work in offices obviously have a harder time getting these types of exercise, so formal exercise like the types previously mentioned are essential to maintain health.

TIP

Taking the stairs, walking to do errands when possible, and taking a stroll after a meal are great ways to get more movement without making major changes in your schedule. You don't need to run a marathon to stay fit. Thirty to 40 minutes of brisk walking, tai chi, yoga, or swimming, for example, when combined with a diet of nutritious foods like those featured in Chapter 15, can cause the tissues and cells in your body to heal and repair themselves.

If you're not used to exercising, choosing the right type can be difficult. Maybe you're out of shape or lack energy due to other physical limitations. If this sounds familiar, don't worry — nowadays there are types of exercise that can benefit everyone, no matter their body type or physical condition. For example, you can try Walk at Home exercise videos; head to www.walkathome.com to learn more. Or go to www.youtube.com/@LeslieSansonesWalkatHome for free videos on YouTube. If walking is challenging for you, you can find chair aerobics videos on YouTube, too — just go to www.youtube.com and search for "chair aerobics."

REMEMBER

If you wait for the ideal time to start exercise, you may never start. By starting where you're at, and letting the exercise be part of your healing routine, you'll be able to improve every day. Starting off short and sweet is better than trying to achieve your desired workout on day one.

TIP

Here are a some tips to ensure that you get enough physical activity every day:

>> Acknowledge the health benefits of exercise, and make it a priority.

>> Choose activities you enjoy so that you'll be more likely to continue doing them.

>> Notice the endorphins! Exercising increases happiness hormones, and when you've established a routine, they'll help motivate you to continue.

>> Exercise outdoors when possible. It increases the psychological benefits of the movement.

Join sports teams or exercise groups/classes to help keep your commitment.

>> Experiment with different types of exercise so you don't get bored.

>> Keep a go-to list of types of exercises you can do within different time slots and schedule them into your calendar. Even ten minutes of exercise is better than none at all, so don't wait to move until you have a full hour free.

REMEMBER

Talk with your doctor before beginning a new exercise regime, especially if your physical condition is compromised or you're afraid that it may be.

Reducing Stress

One of the key ways in which stress may impact cholesterol is through the prolonged activation of the body's "fight-or-flight" response. When you're stressed, the body releases hormones such as cortisol and adrenaline, which help mobilize energy sources, including fats and sugars, to prepare for immediate action. In the short term, this can lead to a rise in circulating fatty acids and lipoproteins, including LDL cholesterol.

Some studies suggest that chronic stress, particularly when combined with unhealthy coping mechanisms such as poor diet or lack of physical activity, may contribute to long-term elevations in LDL and reductions in HDL, the protective cholesterol that helps remove excess fats from the bloodstream. However, the direct link between stress and cholesterol levels is not as firmly established as with other factors like diet and exercise.

Investigations into the effects of workplace strain on cardiovascular health have consistently revealed a connection between job-related pressures and unfavorable lipid profiles. A study involving more than 91,000 working people across diverse occupations indicated that heightened occupational stress correlated with elevated levels of LDL cholesterol and diminished levels of HDL cholesterol. Those experiencing significant work-related strain were more likely to be prescribed cholesterol-lowering medications.

Research focusing on law enforcement personnel in Iowa highlighted that officers, especially women, reported greater stress levels and exhibited higher rates of elevated cholesterol and diabetes compared to other women residing in the state. Notably, female officers experiencing substantial stress were often classified as overweight or obese, with a significant majority attributing their health challenges to the pressures of their profession.

Additional research examining a group of 439 professional drivers, including bus, truck, and taxi operators, demonstrated that those subjected to high levels of job-related stress were more prone to displaying unhealthy lipid levels, including elevated LDL cholesterol and triglycerides, along with reduced HDL cholesterol and increased blood pressure.

A study of 208 college students, assessed blood parameters during examination periods. Findings revealed that these stressful times were associated with increased levels of stress hormones, such as cortisol and adrenaline, and elevated total and LDL cholesterol.

REMEMBER

Approaches to mitigating stress have shown promise in improving lipid profiles. Techniques aimed at reducing stress, such as practicing mindfulness, engaging in meditation, and maintaining regular physical activity, have been associated with both a reduction in harmful LDL cholesterol and an increase in beneficial HDL cholesterol.

In the following sections, we show you how stress affects cholesterol and disease risk and offer strategies for reducing stress.

Seeing how stress affects cholesterol and cardiovascular risk

Stress may contribute to the oxidation of LDL cholesterol, which plays a key role in the development of atherosclerosis. Psychological stress is associated with increased oxidative stress in the body, partly due to the overproduction of free radicals and a reduction in antioxidant defenses. Some animal and human studies suggest that chronic stress can increase oxidative modification of LDL, but more research is needed to fully understand the extent of this effect in different populations. That said, stress reduction strategies such as meditation and mindfulness have been linked to lower oxidative stress markers, which could, in turn, help reduce LDL oxidation and its harmful effects on artery walls.

A clearer connection exists between stress and inflammation, which is a well-established driver of CVD. Chronic stress can lead to prolonged activation of the immune system, increasing levels of inflammatory markers such as CRP and pro-inflammatory cytokines. This inflammatory state contributes to plaque formation in the arteries and can make existing plaques more unstable, raising the risk of heart attack or stroke. Unlike the evidence on stress and cholesterol levels, the relationship between stress and inflammation is more firmly established, and managing stress through relaxation techniques, social support, or lifestyle changes has been shown to reduce inflammatory markers.

Another concerning effect of chronic stress is its impact on blood vessel function. Stress can impair *endothelial function* (the ability of blood vessels to dilate properly), which increases blood pressure and reduces the arteries' flexibility. Over time, this contributes to vascular stiffness and increases the risk of plaque rupture. Additionally, stress-related spikes in blood pressure and heart rate can place additional strain on arterial walls, making them more susceptible to damage and increasing the likelihood of clot formation.

Although the direct effects of stress on cholesterol levels are less well understood than those of exercise, there is strong evidence linking stress to increased inflammation, oxidative stress, and impaired blood vessel function. Managing stress through mindfulness, relaxation techniques, physical activity, and strong social connections has been associated with lower levels of inflammatory markers and improved heart health. Reducing stress alone may not dramatically alter cholesterol levels, but it plays an important role in creating a more resilient cardiovascular system and lowering overall CVD risk.

Managing stress

Stressful events and periods are a normal part of life. No matter how hard you try, you can't completely cancel out stress. There will always be situations in your life that you can't change. The key is to learn strategies you can draw upon to reduce your stress and minimize its effects on your mind and body.

Yoga

Modern yoga therapy combines ancient wisdom practices with modern research. Make sure that your yoga instructor (whether they're live or virtual) is certified to teach. You may choose to work with a yoga therapist who has a degree as well. Yoga therapy can work to indirectly improve overall cardiovascular health through stress reduction and improved blood circulation.

To perform yoga, you'll choose a comfortable space, perform light stretches, practice deep breathing, and perform a variety of poses. The cooldown consists of lying in a specific pose, engaging in deep breathing and perhaps a brief meditation, reflection, and gentle stretching.

ALLOWING YOURSELF TO BE HAPPY

A different approach to stress is to allow yourself a dedicated time to completely acknowledge the pain or discomfort you're feeling. After that time, decide that instead of trying to manage issues that make you feel powerless, you're going to shift your intention to what empowers you. This is tricky for many people because cultural attitudes make us feel guilty for enjoying anything unless everything is perfect. The truth is, life is rarely "perfect," and if you wait for it to be perfect in order to allow yourself to experience joy and happiness, you won't spend much time being happy at all.

Yet being happy can positively impact health. The happier you can allow yourself to become, the better you'll feel and the better your body will respond. The stress can't be as disruptive if you choose to focus on other things as much as possible. This isn't an easy task, but as with physical exercise, you have to start somewhere and even baby steps will produce results. In Italian there is a saying, *"Chi va piano va lontano, eppure sano,"* Which means "Who goes slowly goes far, and does so healthfully."

Recognizing that you're born with the capacity for happiness and joy, and doing what you can to allow yourself to experience these emotions, are crucial not only to "managing stress," but also to overall well-being. Check out the daily habits checklist at the end of this chapter to discover ways to create more happiness and joy in your life. You don't have to wait for everything around you to be "perfect" before giving yourself permission to be happy.

Consistently practicing yoga can improve strength, flexibility, and overall health. If you're new to yoga, you can find introductory videos online, as well as in-person classes and therapists to work with you individually.

TIP

One extremely popular yoga instructor is Adriene Mishler, who runs the Yoga with Adriene YouTube channel (www.youtube.com/yogawithadriene). There you can find yoga videos for beginners (and beyond).

Also, check out the range of *For Dummies* books on yoga, including *Chair Yoga For Dummies* by Larry Payne and Don Henry, *Yoga After 50 For Dummies* by Larry Payne, and *Yoga All-in-One For Dummies* (all published by John Wiley & Sons, Inc.).

Breathwork

The origins of breathwork began with the practice of yoga. Focusing on breath by nourishing your mind and body by inhaling, and releasing toxins and stress by exhaling, is the basis of breathwork. Research suggests that breathwork can potentially help to elevate your mood, have an anti-inflammatory effect on the body, and have an alkalizing effect on your blood's pH. It may also help to regulate the central nervous system during times of stress, balance blood pressure, improve sleep, reduce post-traumatic stress disorder (PTSD), improve immune function, and release stress hormones.

Emotional benefits of breathwork may include increased feelings of contentment, joy, and a positive outlook on life. It may also improve the feelings associated with anxiety and depression, as well as improve mental focus.

There are numerous types of breathwork techniques, including the following:

>> Alternate nostril breathing, which helps to encourage balance between mind and body

>> Deep abdominal breathing, which helps the body relax

>> 4-7-8 breathing, which helps empty the lungs

>> Breath of fire, which helps to provide a sense of steadiness

Some more advanced forms of breathwork require an instructor's assistance.

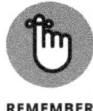
REMEMBER

For maximum results, breathwork takes focus and time to improve techniques. Attempting breathwork while distracted will cause it to be less effective.

TIP

For help getting started, check out *Breathing Exercises For Dummies* by Shamash Alidina (published by John Wiley & Sons, Inc.).

Mindfulness

Mindfulness is a psychological practice that helps to keep you in the present moment. It involves paying attention to the present moment with acceptance and without judgment. It teaches you to be fully aware of your own thoughts, emotions, feelings, and conditions without getting caught up in them. Practicing mindfulness involves setting an intention to focus on the present moment, paying attention to how you feel, and accepting all experiences without judgment.

REMEMBER

Mindful walking, mindful eating, and meditation are all ways to practice mindfulness throughout your day. To incorporate mindfulness into your lifestyle, you can watch videos, read books, or take courses on it. There are health coaches and meditation instructors who teach mindfulness as well.

TIP

Check out *Mindfulness For Dummies* by Shamash Alidina (published by John Wiley & Sons, Inc.).

Although always popular in many traditional cultures and among the spiritual community, meditation is also an effective tool to improve health and happiness. Psychologists have found that mindfulness meditation changes the brain and biology in positive ways, which can lead to improved mental and physical health.

TIP

Headspace (www.headspace.com) is an app that focuses on mindfulness meditation.

The most common types of meditation in the United States currently are:

>> **Guided imagery:** You envision what you'd like to experience, feel the emotions of it, and allow yourself to act as if you are in a movie with your desired outcome taking place.

>> **Mindfulness:** The Buddhist technique mentioned earlier, which helps you to be at peace in the present moment.

>> **Spiritual:** Focuses on developing a deeper understanding of spiritual/religious meaning and connection with a higher power. Jewish Kabbalistic practices, Muslim Sufi Dhikr (remembrance of God) ceremonies, and Christian contemplative prayer are all examples of meditation that can infuse a sense of hope and relieve stress.

>> **Movement:** Combines movement (such as walking) with mindfulness techniques to help you to feel more relaxed, centered, and at peace.

- » **Focused:** Concentrating on something internal, like your breath, or something external like music, prayer beads, healing sounds, and using any of the five senses to help you center and focus your attention.

- » **Transcendental:** This form of meditation is a specific practice designed to quiet the mind and induce a state of calm and peace. It involves the use of mantras and is taught by certified Transcendental Meditation (TM) practitioners in individual or group settings. A large amount of scientific research highlights its effectiveness.

- » **Mantra:** Hindu, Sufi, and Buddhist traditions are among the many that include mantra therapy. It uses a repetitive sound or word, such as *om,* or the names of God to clear the mind and to reach for a desired state of consciousness.

- » **Loving-kindness:** Loving-kindness involves opening the heart, body, and mind to send and receive love from others. In addition to improving compassion and kindness, it can also help people to overcome anger and resentment and to feel as if they've communicated with people who they can't actually speak with.

- » **Progressive relaxation:** Also called body scan meditation, it involves slowly tightening and relaxing one muscle group at a time throughout the body, as well as imagining a gentle wave or type of energy flowing through the body to help you relax and transform physical conditions. It helps to relieve stress before sleeping.

Reduced stress; better sleep; improved emotions, focus, and mood; increased adaptability; healthier aging; and reduced aggression, stress, and blood pressure are all associated with meditating.

Other strategies to unlock happiness

Dopamine, serotonin, oxytocin, and endorphins are hormones nicknamed the "feel-good hormones" because of the happy and, sometimes, euphoric feelings they create. Harnessing the power of "happiness hormones" can also help to reduce stress. Being happy leads to reduced stress and can increase lifespan — happy people tend to have healthier habits and manage stress more effectively than those who are unhappy.

TIP

Table 10-1 lists the feel-good hormones and when they're released.

TABLE 10-1

Increasing the Feel-Good Hormones

Hormone	Nickname	Examples of When It's Released
Dopamine	The "reward hormone"	When you celebrate small victories, enjoy food, participate in self-care activities (see Chapter 9), and complete tasks
Serotonin	The "mood stabilizer"	When you're exposed to sunshine, meditating, running, cycling, or swimming
Oxytocin	The "love hormone"	When you receive physical affection, such as playing with a baby or dog, being affectionate with someone you love, holding hands, hugging, expression and receiving gratitude, and giving and receiving compliments
Endorphins	The "pain killer hormone"	When you're exercising, laughing, experiencing aromatherapy, watching a comedy, or consuming dark chocolate

TIP

Try to incorporate as many of these activities into your day as possible to reduce stress and increase feelings of happiness.

YOUR DAILY HEALTHY HABIT CHECKLIST

Here are some things you can do every day to feel your best and manage stress:

- Get enough sleep.
- Eat a healthful diet.
- Exercise.
- Do yoga.
- Do breathwork.
- Meditate.
- Practice mindfulness.
- Keep a gratitude journal.
- Practice gratitude — spend as much time as possible being truly grateful for what you have.
- Take naps.
- Engage in self-care rituals (see Chapter 9).

- Seek out professional help when you're having trouble coping with an issue on your own.

- Spend time doing activities that you enjoy.

- Spend time outdoors.

- Eat meals with others whenever possible.

- Prioritize socializing with friends and family.

- Learn new activities.

- Listen to healing or soothing music.

- Make your own meals.

- Start or maintain healthful dining rituals with friends and family.

- Aim for 5 to 12 servings of fresh fruits and vegetables daily.

- Let go and transform unhealthful habits.

- Prioritize your own happiness — incorporate activities that increase mood-boosting hormones.

- Spend some time in the sun.

- Play with a baby or pets.

- Hug your loved ones.

- Use aromatherapy.

- Watch comedies.

- Indulge in community activities.

- Keep a positive outlook on life.

4

Incorporating Medicines and Holistic Approaches

Discover drug options for cholesterol.

Identify which drugs are used in managing cholesterol.

Choose the best medicine for you.

Learn how holistic approaches can help.

See how making healthy choices and emotional well-being matter.

Explore complementary therapies and the metaphysical point of view.

Chapter **11**

Evaluating Treatment Options for Cholesterol

You may be reading this book because you're taking cholesterol-lowering medication or because your doctor has talked to you about your lipid panel. You may know someone who is taking a statin or other cholesterol-lowering drug, or have family or friends who have considered medication or brought the topic up in conversation. You've probably come across media articles on the subject and seen ads for various drugs on TV.

In this chapter, we explain when medications may be appropriate, the different drug options, and how to find the right option for you. We also cover other treatments for cardiovascular disease (CVD), so you have a full picture. This chapter will help you make your own decision about your cholesterol management and enable you to have fruitful conversations with your doctor.

Knowing When Medications Are Considered for High Cholesterol

There are usually four circumstances in which a person may end up taking cholesterol-lowering medications:

>> Secondary prevention following a diagnosis of CVD with symptoms

>> Secondary prevention following the discovery of CVD without symptoms

>> Primary prevention of CVD with very high risk

>> Primary prevention of CVD with moderately increased risk

Each of these situations needs a different approach to cholesterol management, though the treatment itself may be similar. In the following sections, we cover both secondary prevention and primary prevention.

Secondary prevention

For secondary prevention, the goal is to prevent more cardiovascular events in people who have already experienced them or have warning symptoms. For people who have a history of atherosclerosis, a fundamental strategy to prevent the worsening of CVD is statins. The use of statins in this situation is grounded in substantial scientific evidence.

For example, a person who has symptoms of *angina* (chest pain from reduced blood supply to the heart) or who has had a heart attack is at high risk of further events and complications unless the atherosclerotic plaque formation and rupture is inhibited.

CVD doesn't just compromise the blood vessels of the heart — it can present through a range of symptoms, reflecting the varied impact on the circulatory system. For example, angina, palpitations, and dizziness can indicate underlying heart conditions, which may be a result of atherosclerosis of the coronary arteries. Someone experiencing transient ischemic attacks (TIAs) may have temporary neurological deficits, such as weakness or speech difficulties, which serve as warnings of potential strokes. Similarly, peripheral artery disease (PAD) causes symptoms like *claudication* (in which leg pain occurs during exertion) or in severe cases, *limb ischemia* (harmful insufficient blood flow to a limb), showing how CVD can affect blood flow to the extremities with significant consequences.

The primary role of treatment is to lower low-density lipoprotein (LDL) cholesterol in atherosclerosis, and inhibit the process in which plaque accumulates within artery walls, leading to heart attacks and strokes. Statins function by inhibiting an enzyme in the liver that produces cholesterol, thereby significantly lowering LDL levels. They also have a role in preventing oxidation of LDL, plaque inflammation, and rupture.

Statins are strongly recommended for people with established CVD, including those with a history of heart attacks, stroke, TIA, PAD, or coronary artery disease. A pivotal study supporting this practice was the Scandinavian Simvastatin Survival Study (4S). This landmark trial published in 1994 in the *Lancet* demonstrated a significant reduction in total mortality, coronary heart disease mortality, and major coronary events in patients with coronary heart disease and elevated cholesterol when treated with simvastatin. Other significant studies, such as the Cholesterol and Recurrent Events (CARE) and Long-term Intervention with Pravastatin in Ischemic Heart Disease (LIPID) trials, have further reinforced the benefits of statin therapy in secondary prevention. Current clinical guidelines reflect this robust body of evidence, emphasizing the importance of statin therapy for secondary prevention, often recommending high-intensity statins to achieve substantial LDL cholesterol reduction.

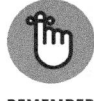
REMEMBER

Statins are recommended for secondary prevention of CVD. There is a general consensus that they're beneficial regardless of initial LDL cholesterol levels. It may seem strange that a person without a diagnosis of CVD may be advised that their cholesterol levels are acceptable, but very soon afterward may unexpectedly develop angina. They'll then be advised that their cholesterol must be aggressively lowered (with an accompanying unmeasured reduction in LDL oxidation and inflammation) using a statin.

Although statins remain the cornerstone of cholesterol management, other medications play a role, particularly when statins are not tolerated or when additional LDL reduction is needed. Ezetimibe works by inhibiting cholesterol absorption in the intestines, and PCSK9 inhibitors enhance the liver's ability to remove LDL cholesterol from the bloodstream. Bile acid sequestrants bind to bile acids in the gut, promoting their excretion and lowering cholesterol levels. We cover these drugs in more detail later in this chapter, but the evidence supporting the effects of these alternative medications — specifically regarding plaque stabilization, LDL oxidation, and inflammation reduction — is generally less extensive than it is for statins.

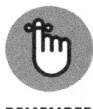
REMEMBER

The choice of therapy should be guided by a comprehensive assessment of your individual risk factors, tolerability, and specific lipid abnormalities, always prioritizing statin use when possible due to the strong evidence supporting their efficacy and safety.

The use of statins in secondary prevention is also recommended when a person is found to have CVD during screening or when it's a coincidental finding from other medical investigations or interventions. For example, a person may have an EKG in preparation for a surgical operation, and the EKG may suggest they have heart disease. A routine blood test may reveal kidney disease due to reduced blood flow from atherosclerosis in the major arteries supplying the kidneys. A specialist may be undertaking a liver scan and discover an abnormality of the *aorta* (the main artery in the abdomen). These and other conditions may be detected in a person who has developed CVD but not yet experienced symptoms.

Primary prevention

In Chapters 7 and 8, we explore the risk tools used to asses a person's likelihood of developing CVD when they have no history suggesting existing significant disease. The risk algorithm is based on several factors, including cholesterol level, and provides the estimated chance of a person developing CVD in the next ten years.

The various risk tools have different criteria. Some, but not all, tools include conditions that tend to significantly increase the risk of CVD:

>> **Diabetes:** Diabetes, particularly type 2 diabetes, significantly elevates the risk of CVD, making statin therapy a common preventive measure regardless of baseline cholesterol levels. The presence of diabetes itself is considered a major risk factor, justifying the routine use of statins to reduce this heightened risk.

>> **Chronic kidney disease (CKD):** CKD is associated with an increased risk of cardiovascular events, and statins are often recommended to reduce this risk, even in the absence of traditional CVD risk factors.

>> **Familial hypercholesterolemia (FH):** Even without established heart disease, FH necessitates statin therapy, especially when other risk factors are present. A significantly elevated lipoprotein(a) level is recognized as an independent risk factor for CVD as well. Although statins may not directly lower lipoprotein(a), they can still reduce overall cardiovascular risk by lowering LDL cholesterol, particularly when accompanied by other risk factors (see Chapter 2).

>> **Inflammatory autoimmune conditions:** These conditions, like rheumatoid arthritis, lupus, and psoriasis, are associated with chronic inflammation, which contributes to an increased risk of atherosclerosis and cardiovascular events. The chronic inflammatory state present in these conditions accelerates the development of plaques and, therefore, the risk of a cardiovascular event. In these cases, statins are used to address the elevated cardiovascular risk stemming from the chronic inflammation inherent in these autoimmune disorders.

REMEMBER

In any of these situations, the decision to initiate statin therapy is guided by a comprehensive assessment of your overall risk profile.

Surveying the Medications Used to Treat High Cholesterol

Cholesterol medications work through several key mechanisms to lower cholesterol levels and reduce cardiovascular risk. Some drugs target cholesterol production by inhibiting enzymes involved in its production, leading to lower levels of circulating LDL cholesterol. Others block cholesterol absorption in the intestine, preventing dietary cholesterol from entering the bloodstream and reducing overall levels. Another approach involves increasing cholesterol removal from the body, often by enhancing the liver's ability to clear LDL cholesterol from circulation. Beyond these well-established mechanisms, there is ongoing research into the additional benefits of cholesterol-lowering therapies, including their potential role in reducing oxidative stress and inflammation, improving endothelial function, and stabilizing atherosclerotic plaques. Although these effects are not fully understood, they may contribute to the broader cardiovascular benefits observed with cholesterol-lowering treatments beyond their impact on lipid levels alone.

The decision about which medication to choose depends on several factors. The most widely prescribed drugs are statins, because the evidence in support of their effectiveness is very well established. Other medications may be used in specific circumstances (for example, if a statin is not tolerated because of side effects, if it's contraindicated in the first place, or if you need more than one drug to achieve the target cholesterol level).

REMEMBER

Decisions about medications should involve a discussion about the potential benefits of any given level of cholesterol and CVD risk, whether lifestyle modifications should be tried first, the possibility of harm from side effects, as well as your personal preferences and values.

In the following sections, we offer a broad overview of the most commonly used medications to treat cholesterol. Discuss the details of your drugs with your doctor and read the patient information leaflet that's supplied with the medication for more information.

Statins

Statins are the most commonly prescribed medications for lowering cholesterol, particularly LDL cholesterol. Statins work by inhibiting an enzyme called HMG-CoA reductase, which plays a critical role in cholesterol production within the liver. By blocking this enzyme, the liver produces less cholesterol and, as a result, increases its uptake of LDL cholesterol from the bloodstream, leading to an overall reduction in LDL levels. Statins also offer additional benefits, such as reducing inflammation in blood vessels and stabilizing plaques, which can help prevent heart attacks.

Different statins vary in their potency and how long they remain active in the body. Atorvastatin and rosuvastatin are considered more potent and long-acting, while others like simvastatin and pravastatin are less powerful. Statins are typically taken once a day, with some requiring evening dosing because cholesterol production is highest at night.

Many people tolerate statins well, but some experience muscle pain, fatigue, or mild digestive issues. Muscle-related symptoms can often be managed by switching to a different statin or adjusting the dose. In rare cases, statins can cause severe muscle damage (a condition called *rhabdomyolysis*), leading to muscle breakdown and potential kidney damage because of circulating protein overload. They may also slightly increase the risk of new-onset diabetes, particularly in those with preexisting risk factors. Liver enzyme elevations can occur, although serious liver damage is rare.

Statins can interact with certain medications, including some antibiotics and antifungal drugs, increasing the risk of side effects. Grapefruit juice can interfere with the metabolism of some statins, leading to higher drug levels in the blood.

Cholesterol absorption inhibitors

Cholesterol absorption inhibitors, such as ezetimibe, lower cholesterol by preventing its absorption from food and bile in the intestines. Ezetimibe works by blocking a protein called NPC1L1 in the small intestine, which is responsible for absorbing cholesterol from food and bile. By reducing the amount of cholesterol entering the bloodstream, the liver compensates by taking up more LDL cholesterol, lowering overall levels. Ezetimibe is often prescribed alongside statins for added cholesterol reduction, especially in people who do not achieve their target LDL levels with statins alone.

Ezetimibe is generally well tolerated, but some people may experience stomach pain, diarrhea, or fatigue. Rare but potentially more serious side effects include liver enzyme elevation and muscle pain, particularly when combined with statins.

Bile acid sequestrants

Bile acid sequestrants lower cholesterol by binding to bile acids in the gut, forcing the liver to use more cholesterol to make new bile acids. Bile acids are essential for digesting fats, and they're normally recycled by the body. Bile acid sequestrants, such as cholestyramine and colesevelam, bind to bile acids in the intestines, preventing their reabsorption. As a result, the liver uses more cholesterol to make new bile acids, lowering LDL cholesterol in the bloodstream. These drugs are particularly useful for people who can't tolerate statins. However, they can interfere with the absorption of fat-soluble vitamins (A, D, E, and K) and other medications.

The most common side effects are constipation, bloating, and gas. Increasing fiber intake and drinking plenty of water can help. In rare cases, bile acid sequestrants may contribute to gallstone formation or affect blood clotting due to reduced vitamin K absorption.

Fibrates

Fibrates are mainly used to lower triglycerides and raise high-density lipoprotein (HDL) cholesterol, instead of significantly lowering LDL cholesterol. Fibrates, such as fenofibrate and gemfibrozil, activate a receptor called PPAR-alpha in the liver. This increases the breakdown of triglycerides and enhances the removal of particles that carry cholesterol in the blood. These drugs are highly effective at lowering triglycerides, which can be important for preventing pancreatitis in people who have high triglycerides. They also modestly increase HDL cholesterol, though their impact on heart disease risk is less clear.

Fibrates can cause digestive issues, muscle pain, and an increased risk of gallstones. When combined with statins, the risk of muscle damage is significantly higher.

Niacin

Niacin, or nicotinic acid, was once a mainstay of cholesterol treatment but today it's used less frequently due to side effects and limited evidence of additional benefit. Niacin reduces the liver's production of LDL and very-low-density lipoprotein (VLDL) cholesterol while increasing HDL cholesterol. It can lower LDL and triglycerides and significantly raise HDL. However, recent studies suggest it may not provide significant additional heart benefits beyond statins.

Flushing (a warm, red sensation on the skin) is a common side effect, but taking aspirin before niacin can help. High doses may increase the risk of liver damage, gout, and blood glucose elevation.

PCSK9 inhibitors

PCSK9 inhibitors are a newer class of cholesterol-lowering drugs, particularly useful for high-risk patients. (PCSK9 is short for *proprotein convertase subtilisin/kexin type 9* — hence, the shortened version.) These injectable drugs block PCSK9, a protein that degrades LDL receptors in the liver. By inhibiting PCSK9, the liver is able to remove more LDL cholesterol from the blood. By influencing oxidized LDL uptake and inflammation, PCSK9 inhibitors may also contribute to plaque stabilization. A stable plaque is less likely to rupture, and ruptures can cause a heart attack or stroke. Like statins, PCSK9 inhibitors may have benefits beyond just LDL-cholesterol lowering. They're given as an injection every two to four weeks and are extremely effective, particularly for those with FH or statin intolerance.

PCSK9 inhibitors are generally well tolerated, but they may cause injection-site reactions, flu-like symptoms, and, rarely, neurocognitive effects like memory issues.

MTP inhibitors

Microsomal triglyceride transfer protein (MTP) inhibitors, such as lomitapide, are specialized drugs for severe cholesterol disorders. MTP inhibitors are primarily used for a very specific and relatively rare condition, homozygous FH, which is a severe genetic disorder that causes extremely high levels of LDL cholesterol. They inhibit a liver protein that is essential for making LDL cholesterol.

They can cause significant gastrointestinal symptoms and liver enzyme elevations, requiring careful monitoring. Their complex effects are still being understood by researchers.

ACL inhibitors

ATP-citrate lyase (ACL) inhibitors, such as bempedoic acid, are an alternative for people who can't tolerate statins. They work upstream of statins in the cholesterol synthesis pathway. Bempedoic acid is a relatively newer medication compared to statins, which have been used for decades. Therefore, there's less long-term data and clinical experience available. Clinical trials have demonstrated its effectiveness in lowering LDL cholesterol, but ongoing research continues to explore its long-term effects and potential benefits. Until there is convincing evidence not only of reducing cholesterol but also preventing CVD, their use will be limited.

ACL inhibitors may increase uric acid levels and cause joint pain.

WHAT ABOUT STANOLS AND STEROLS?

Plant stanols and sterols (described in Chapter 5), can be found in fortified foods as well as the natural foods where they occur. They lower LDL cholesterol by blocking its absorption in the gut, but they're not regarded as a primary treatment and their impact on cardiovascular events is debated. Although they're effective for cholesterol reduction at recommended doses (2 to 3 grams per day), exceeding this may interfere with vitamin absorption, and those with *sitosterolemia* (a rare condition covered in Chapter 3) should avoid them entirely. They're often added to margarine and other ultra-processed spreads where it's quite difficult to know the "dose" you're getting and how the other ingredients may be affecting your metabolism.

It's probably better to stick to natural sources of stanols where they're part of the food matrix, and add extra-virgin olive oil instead of using an artificially produced margarine.

Omega-3 fatty acids

Omega-3 fatty acids, whether from your diet or a prescription, can be helpful for lipid regulation (see Chapter 5). In prescription form, they're mainly used to lower triglycerides. Prescription omega-3s, like icosapent ethyl (Vascepa), have also been shown to reduce the risk of heart problems.

The key distinction from dietary omega-3s is that prescription omega-3s are in the form of a concentrated medicine, giving a specific, high dose of the most beneficial part of the omega-3s, while omega-3s from food provide a wider range of these healthy fats, but in smaller and less controlled amounts.

Omega-3s can cause burping and upset stomach. In high doses, they may increase the risk of bleeding.

Personalizing Therapy

Decisions about which medications to use and when to introduce or change them depend on several factors, including the initial results of the lipid panel, the risk reduction goals, and other aspects, including your lifestyle. Your doctor will consider the strength of evidence of the benefits of a therapy in a particular circumstance and its side effect profile. The final decisions should be part of an agreed plan to best manage your cholesterol, focused on the desired outcome — reducing the risk of CVD as opposed to "treating numbers" or test results.

Considering targets and dosing

The medications you take, as well as their doses, will be influenced by the evidence from population data, as well as tailored for you. Your doctor should talk with you and recommend therapy using the best available guidance.

In secondary prevention (for example, if you've already had a heart attack, stroke, or other cardiovascular event), the goal is to lower LDL cholesterol as much as possible to reduce the risk of future problems. Medical guidelines from organizations like the American Heart Association (AHA), the European Society of Cardiology (ESC), and the National Institute for Health and Care Excellence (NICE) all emphasize aggressive LDL lowering in these high-risk patients. NICE, for example, typically recommends aiming for LDL levels below 2.0 mmol/L (77.3 mg/dL), while the ESC suggests an even lower target of 1.4 mmol/L (38.67 mg/dL) for those at the highest risk. The AHA doesn't specify a hard numerical target but strongly advises using high-intensity statins as the first line of treatment and adding other medications if needed to achieve sufficient LDL reduction.

For secondary prevention, the treatment process usually follows a structured approach. First, your doctor will prescribe a high-intensity statin, such as atorvastatin or rosuvastatin, to lower LDL production as much as possible. If your LDL levels remain above the recommended target despite the maximum tolerated dose of a statin, the next step is typically adding ezetimibe to block cholesterol absorption in the small intestine. If further lowering is required, PCSK9 inhibitors, such as alirocumab or evolocumab, may be introduced to further clear LDL cholesterol from the bloodstream. Because PCSK9 inhibitors are expensive, their use is often reserved for patients at the highest risk, under specialist care, or those who do not achieve sufficient LDL lowering with other treatments. Physicians carefully monitor how well each patient responds to treatment, adjusting medications as necessary to keep LDL as low as possible.

For primary prevention, where the goal is to prevent CVD before it happens, the approach is more personalized. Instead of focusing strictly on LDL targets, treatment is guided by an individual's overall risk of developing CVD in the next ten years. Doctors use risk calculators, such as those explained in Chapter 7 and 8, to estimate this risk based on factors like age, blood pressure, cholesterol levels, smoking status, and medical history. If your risk is above a certain threshold — usually 10 percent or higher over ten years — guidelines typically recommend discussing starting statin therapy. There are however very real limitations of these risk tools (see Chapter 8).

The intensity of statin treatment depends on the level of risk. Moderate-risk individuals may start with a moderate-intensity statin, while those at higher risk (such as people with diabetes or FH) are more likely to be prescribed a high-intensity statin right away. NICE provides numerical LDL targets even in primary prevention, while the AHA focuses more on ensuring that patients receive the right intensity of statin therapy rather than reaching a specific LDL number. If LDL levels remain high despite statin use, doctors may increase the dose or switch to a more potent statin. In some cases, other cholesterol-lowering medications, such as bile acid sequestrants or fibrates, may be considered, although these are used less often in primary prevention because the evidence in CVD prevention is not well established despite their ability to reduce LDL cholesterol. Patients who can't tolerate statins may also be given alternative treatments.

LDL targets play a crucial role in high-risk cases, but not everyone requires strict cholesterol monitoring. In some situations, doctors may prescribe statins without frequently checking LDL levels, particularly in moderate-risk individuals where the primary goal is simply to reduce overall cardiovascular risk rather than hit a specific cholesterol number. This approach is often used in older adults or people who may find regular cholesterol tests inconvenient or stressful. In these cases, the emphasis is on ensuring patients take their medications consistently.

Across different countries, guidelines for managing cholesterol can vary slightly. The ESC, NICE, and AHA all provide expert recommendations, but the specific LDL targets, risk thresholds, and treatment approaches may differ. Other regions, such as Australia and New Zealand, also have their own guidelines, which generally follow similar principles but sometimes use different numerical thresholds or targets. Despite these variations, the overall strategy remains the same: people at higher risk of CVD recommended to have more intensive LDL lowering, while those at moderate risk are treated based more on an individualized assessment with weighing of benefits against possible disadvantages of taking medications.

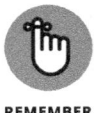

REMEMBER

Ultimately, doctors, in discussion with their patients, balance the need for effective cholesterol management with practical considerations, ensuring that each receives the most appropriate level of treatment based on their personal risk factors, health status, and ability to tolerate medications.

Knowing how low to go

The general principle guiding statin use especially in secondary CVD prevention is that they're beneficial regardless of initial LDL cholesterol levels, whereas in primary prevention the aim is to reduce high levels as part of risk management. However, the concept of "how low is too low" remains a subject of ongoing discussion and evolving clinical practice. The primary goal in secondary prevention is to minimize cardiovascular risk, and statins have consistently demonstrated their effectiveness in achieving this goal. Modern guidelines emphasize the importance of lowering LDL cholesterol to very low levels, particularly for very high-risk patients. A growing body of evidence supports the notion that "lower is better" when it comes to LDL cholesterol levels in secondary prevention, leading clinicians to favor aggressive LDL lowering, especially in high-risk individuals.

Clinical decision-making, however, must be individualized, taking into account factors such as patient age, *comorbidities* (other medical conditions), potential drug interactions, and tolerability. Very low LDL values are becoming increasingly common, but physicians carefully weigh the risks and benefits of further lowering in each particular patient.

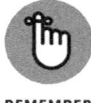

REMEMBER

Cholesterol serves a purpose in the body including building cell membranes, producing hormones and helping absorption of some nutrients. High levels of cholesterol, oxidative stress, and chronic inflammation are often associated with lifestyle choices, so it's important to reduce the risk of CVD, but it's also crucial that research continues to explore the effects of cholesterol reduction on its function and role especially as we age.

Watching for drug interactions

Many people who take one or more medications for cholesterol may also be taking other drugs, perhaps for blood pressure, diabetes, or kidney disease, which are commonly associated with an increased risk of CVD.

We can't list all the potential interactions between the numerous drugs you may be prescribed, but it's important that you, your doctors, and other health professionals including pharmacists are aware of the possibility of drugs interfering with each other. The ways in which interactions can occur are numerous. One drug may decrease or increase the concentration or potency of another by affecting its absorption or metabolism. Alternatively, a medication may add to side effects of another or even result in a new adverse reaction altogether, which may occur with neither medication alone but appear when they're used in combination.

REMEMBER

Some medications can be affected by foods. An example of this is the interference of grapefruit juice with statin metabolism.

TIP

If you're taking medications, especially different drugs for different conditions, it's always useful to have the list available for reference and discussion with a health professional, even if you're just purchasing something simple like a cold or flu remedy.

Monitoring treatment and side effects

If you're taking medications for your cholesterol management, have regular reviews with your doctor. This may include physical checks such as blood pressure monitoring or even more detailed assessments of your CVD risk with investigations like an EKG.

You should be given the time to discuss the effects of the drug(s) and any concerns you may have about potential risks or side effects. You should definitely tell your doctor if you've stopped the medications and, if so, for what reason.

You'll likely have regular blood tests to measure your lipids, especially if there are target levels to be achieved and maintained. You may also have liver and kidney function tests to make sure that a medication is not adversely affecting these organs, as well as a diabetes blood test because there is a small chance that statins may increase the risk of developing diabetes.

TIP

Every review is an opportunity to discuss your lifestyle and how you may enjoy an even healthier way of living, whether it's with an excellent diet, exercise, or other aspects like your sleep and well-being.

FUTURE RESEARCH AND DEVELOPMENTS

The direction of further developments in cholesterol-lowering therapies is focused on addressing questions about the efficacy of medications in achieving reductions in CVD outcomes instead of just lowering cholesterol. There are weaknesses in evidence about the benefits, or potential hazards, of treating people aggressively later in life and the long-term effects of some of the newer therapies. There are certainly limitations in the risk reduction algorithms. Although these calculators are becoming more sensitive to the individual, it's important that treatments are considered with more emphasis and inclusion of the effects of lifestyle modification on CVD risk with measurement of more sophisticated markers of inflammation and oxidative stress.

In cholesterol management, new approaches are being developed for people with specific risk factors, such as elevated lipoprotein(a). Gene therapy, which involves modifying or replacing faulty genes to treat or prevent disease, may become a more widely available option in the future.

Looking at Other Common Treatments for Cardiovascular Disease

If extensive atherosclerosis is diagnosed and the buildup of plaque in the arteries is measured, lowering cholesterol alone may not be enough to address the damage already done. Treatment then shifts toward managing the complications of narrowed or blocked arteries, preventing serious events like heart attacks and strokes, and improving blood flow to affected organs. Depending on the severity and location of the disease, different medical and surgical interventions may be necessary.

We summarize these interventions here, because if you're receiving cholesterol-managing medications, you may have experienced some of these therapies for CVD. You can find out more in *Preventing & Reversing Heart Disease For Dummies*, by James M. Rippe, MD (John Wiley & Sons, Inc.).

REMEMBER

Positive lifestyle changes are even more important if you have a diagnosis of atherosclerosis resulting in CVD. It's never too late to enjoy a healthier way of life, and treatments will be much more effective if you're working toward healthier goals.

Surgical interventions

For people experiencing an acute cardiovascular event, such as a heart attack or stroke, emergency procedures can be lifesaving. A common intervention for heart attacks is percutaneous coronary intervention (PCI), commonly known as angioplasty, where a small balloon is used to widen a blocked artery, often followed by the placement of a stent to keep it open.

In cases of severe coronary artery disease, where multiple arteries are affected, coronary artery bypass grafting (CABG), commonly known as bypass surgery, may be performed. In CABG, a healthy blood vessel from another part of the body is used to bypass the blockage and restore blood flow to the heart.

For strokes caused by blood clots, a procedure called mechanical thrombectomy can be performed to physically remove the clot and restore circulation to the brain, reducing the risk of permanent damage.

For chronic conditions, where blood flow is gradually becoming more restricted, planned interventions may be used to improve circulation and prevent worsening symptoms. In peripheral artery disease (PAD), which affects the blood supply to the legs, procedures like angioplasty or bypass surgery can help restore adequate circulation and relieve symptoms such as pain and difficulty walking. In some cases, carotid endarterectomy, a surgical procedure to remove plaque buildup from the carotid arteries in the neck, may be recommended to reduce stroke risk.

Other common treatments for CVD

In addition to surgical treatments, atherosclerosis is often managed with medications that complement cholesterol-lowering therapies. Anticoagulants and antiplatelet drugs, such as aspirin or clopidogrel, help prevent the formation of dangerous blood clots that could block arteries and trigger a heart attack or stroke. Vasodilators, such as nitrates, work by relaxing and widening blood vessels, improving blood flow and reducing symptoms like angina. Blood pressure-lowering medications, including angiotensin-converting enzyme (ACE) inhibitors, beta-blockers, and calcium channel blockers, are commonly used to reduce strain on the heart and slow the progression of artery damage.

These treatments work together to manage atherosclerosis, not just by reducing cholesterol but also by addressing the broader effects of plaque buildup, improving circulation, and lowering the risk of serious cardiovascular events. With the right combination of lifestyle changes, medications, and medical procedures, people with atherosclerosis can significantly improve their health and quality of life.

Chapter **12**

Choosing a Holistic Approach

I n addition to general self-care techniques such as sleep, connection, exercise, diet, and the drug options available to help you manage cholesterol, adopting a holistic approach to your healthcare can enable you to achieve your health goals.

In this chapter, we cover additional healthy lifestyle choices you can make, emotional well-being, complementary therapies, supplements, and even the metaphysical approach to managing cholesterol.

Holistic Approaches

According to *holistic* medical philosophies, everyone has the innate ability to heal. From the holistic viewpoint, a person's illness is a warning sign to address a deeper emotional issue, resistance, or blockage, which the patient is ready to let go of. Holistic health practitioners search for the underlying causes of illness and treat those causes to heal and prevent disease (which they often refer to as "dis-ease") in the body. Sometimes natural medicines such as herbs or supplements are recommended during these types of treatment, but not always.

Nowadays it's very common for holistic practitioners to collaborate with conventional doctors to best address the needs of their patients.

Integrative medical practitioners often combine both conventional and holistic medicine in their practices to best meet the needs of their patients.

Positive lifestyle choices may have a trickle-down effect on your cholesterol levels. They may not "lower bad cholesterol," but if they improve your overall health and lead to a reduction in oxidative stress, they're worth your while.

Here are some lifestyle choices that can help you feel your best daily:

>> Maintaining the best eating plan possible (see Chapters 6, 14, 15, and 17)

>> Getting enough sleep (see Chapter 9)

>> Enjoying connection with others as much as possible (see Chapter 9)

>> Getting exercise and getting outdoors often (see Chapter 10)

>> If necessary, discussing the best supplements and/or drug options for cholesterol with your doctor (see Chapter 11)

>> Consulting an integrative physician or a holistic practitioner who is certified and has an advanced degree in their field

By creating a healthy lifestyle and gradually putting together a medical team that works for you, you'll be able to live your best life regardless of your diagnosis. Because problems with high cholesterol are usually combined with other issues, these types of healthful choices are the best solution for whole-body health.

Find a qualified and regulated practitioner to advise you about complementary therapy. Holistic approaches should not *replace* a conventional approach to management of your medical problems, and they should always be undertaken in discussion with your team of healthcare professionals.

FOCUSING ON YOUR EMOTIONAL WELL-BEING

You are more than your body and your brain. You're a system of energy and consciousness, and your state of consciousness determines how you feel and how your brain and body responds. Emotional well-being is a necessity for overall health because it influences both physical and mental states, as well as daily performance and relationships

Holistic practitioners believe that happiness, along with good health, are the natural state. If anything is hindering your emotional health, it's important to address those issues in order to improve your physical health. As simplistic as it may sound, it wouldn't be an exaggeration to say that many adults have never learned to understand, manage, and express emotions properly. The good news is, it's never too late to improve. Unresolved emotional stressors can contribute to health issues such as heart disease, weakened immune systems, elevated blood pressure, hormonal imbalances, and digestive issues, just to name a few. Having chronic health issues alone can also negatively affect your emotional state.

If you have emotional issues that you'd like help addressing, seek out experts who can help you to create constructive ways of identifying, expressing, and even transforming what you're feeling.

The healthy lifestyle changes listed in this chapter have positive benefits to emotional well-being. Yoga, breathwork, and meditation are also very helpful. Therapy may also help you learn to process your emotions. A health coach may be able to help you sort out your objectives and which type of therapy could be most beneficial.

Complementary Therapies

Complementary therapies, used alone or in addition to others, can increase quality of life, improve well-being, and help you manage your medical symptoms. By definition, they work alongside conventional medicine to support many aspects of health, which is why they're said to *complement* the modern medical approach.

Sometimes it's difficult to find evidence linking the practice of these techniques with measurable outcomes, including benefits for cholesterol management. Some research has been published in peer-reviewed journals but the lack of standardized methods and small numbers of subjects in such trials often make it hard to draw conclusions.

TECHNICAL STUFF

One of the reasons it's difficult to measure the effectiveness of complementary therapies is because they're usually done in conjunction with other types of conventional and complementary therapies. Someone who sees a Reiki practitioner, for example, may also be taking medication, or attending mind-body therapy sessions, so it's difficult to measure which modality is causing the change. Another reason it's challenging to study complementary therapies is because they're uniquely tailored to the needs of the individual. Unlike administering a certain pill to thousands of people, complementary therapies create individual plans that complement the other lifestyle and medical measures a person is using.

It is believed that at least one in five American adults uses mind-body therapy as a form of self-care and to assist them in treating medical conditions. The use of complementary therapies has been consistently on the rise in the United States since the 1990s. In fact, many established U.S. universities offer degrees and certificates in complementary therapies, while others have opened entire schools dedicated to integrative medicine. Several U.S. hospitals are prescribing complementary therapies and mind-body therapy to various groups of patients. If you're having difficulty finding a qualified mind-body practitioner in your area, consult your doctor or look to these hospitals and universities for recommendations.

In the following sections, we cover some commonly used complementary therapies you may try as part of your cholesterol management and general wellness program. You may want to incorporate one or several of these types of therapies into your lifestyle in order to achieve your health goals.

REMEMBER

Whenever beginning a new type of therapy, remember to allow a few weeks to a month to notice their effect before incorporating additional styles. This way, you'll be able to identify how your body responds to each one.

Acupuncture

Acupuncture is a traditional Chinese medicine practice that involves inserting thin needles into specific points on the body to stimulate the body's flow of energy. In traditional Chinese medicine, high cholesterol may be viewed as a result of "qi stagnation" or "phlegm and dampness" accumulation. With the administering of acupuncture, the body's energy circulation is improved to help cholesterol levels.

TECHNICAL STUFF

Qi (pronounced chee) is the name of the vital life force that flows through the body along specific pathways in Traditional Chinese Medicine.

Several small studies and pilot trials suggest that acupuncture may help improve lipid profiles by lowering total cholesterol, low-density lipoprotein (LDL) cholesterol, and triglycerides, while possibly raising high-density lipoprotein (HDL) cholesterol. One theory is that acupuncture may influence the autonomic nervous system, reduce inflammation, and improve liver metabolism, all of which could help your body manage fats more efficiently.

A 2015 meta-analysis of 13 randomized controlled trials found that acupuncture had a positive effect on cholesterol levels, though the studies included were generally small and varied widely in quality.

Acupuncture can positively impact blood lipid levels and insulin resistance, which can help you to manage your cholesterol levels better. We recommend consulting a qualified and certified practitioner in your area who will discuss your medications and underlying medical conditions with you. They may recommend diet and lifestyle changes, as well as supplements, to improve the efficacy of the treatment.

Emotional Freedom Technique (also known as tapping)

Like acupuncture, *Emotional Freedom Technique* (EFT), also known as *tapping,* is a complementary therapy that involves relieving the distress of certain acupressure points on the body. Unlike acupuncture, which requires a practitioner and needles, EFT involves gently tapping on specific points on the body while focusing on negative emotions that you want to transform. EFT is said to work by releasing emotional blockages, and proponents believe that EFT can help the brain "rewire" itself, reducing stressful emotions and negative stimuli.

There is no direct evidence suggesting that EFT can directly influence cholesterol levels, but studies do show that EFT can reduce stress and improve mood, which may indirectly assist in managing stress hormones like cortisol, which may in turn support the management of high cholesterol.

If you're interested in this type of therapy, you can look for a certified EFT practitioner in your area. There are also many videos available online that show you how to tap effectively. Brad Yates is a respected source; check him out at www.youtube.com/@tapwithbrad.

Reiki

Reiki (pronounced *ray*-key) originated in Japan more than a century ago. Reiki is a form of energy medicine or biofield therapy that reduces stress and promotes healing. It's delivered by laying hands on the patient in person or remotely. Reiki is a form of complementary therapy that channels energy to promote relaxation and stress reduction. Reduced stress can lead to an improved mood, better metabolism, a lower heart rate, and lower blood pressure. Reiki may indirectly influence cholesterol through stress reduction and other physiological changes.

Some U.S. hospitals, medical clinics, and hospice centers offer Reiki as a part of treatment. If you seek out the care of a professional on your own, make sure that they have several years of experience. If you're new to Reiki, ask the practitioners how the process works and what you can expect prior to your visit.

Supplements

Several supplements are associated with lowering cholesterol levels. Before adding any supplement to your routine, talk with your doctor about possible contraindications with any medical conditions you may have or interference with any medicines you may be taking.

REMEMBER Regulation of the supplement market is generally not as strong as that of the food and pharmaceutical industry.

REMEMBER For maximum efficacy, make sure you're eating well, exercising, and following all the healthy lifestyle practices mentioned in this book while adding supplements to your routine. No supplement will let you get away with an unhealthy lifestyle.

Here are the supplements that are most commonly used in managing cholesterol:

>> **Bergamot:** Bergamot is a citrus fruit that hails from Calabria, Italy. Supplements made from bergamot are becoming especially popular with those who can't take statins. Some studies suggest that bergamot extract may help reduce total cholesterol, LDL cholesterol, and triglycerides.

>> **Berberine:** Berberine is a natural compound found in some plants like European barberry, goldenseal, goldthread, Oregon grape, and tree turmeric. It may reduce LDL cholesterol.

>> **Fish oil:** Fish oil supplements contain omega-3 fatty acids such as eicosapentaenoic acid (EPA) and docosahexaenoic acid (DHA) and may reduce triglycerides.

>> **Ground flaxseeds:** Flaxseeds may reduce LDL cholesterol. You can add ground flaxseeds to baked goods, smoothies, and yogurt.

>> **Green tea and green tea extract:** Green tea and its concentrated form, green tea extract, which is available in supplement form, may reduce LDL cholesterol.

Metaphysical healing

Metaphysical healing includes approaches that look beyond the physical symptoms of illness to explore their emotional, energetic, or spiritual causes. These methods often include practices like affirmations, energy healing, or chakra balancing, and they're used as complementary tools in parallel with conventional medical treatments.

Chakras are the body's energy centers. In various spiritual and yogic practices, it is believed that balancing the seven chakras of the body leads to physical, mental, and spiritual harmony.

Metaphysical approaches explore the emotional, energetic, and vibrational aspects of illness to identify its root causes — in contrast with conventional Western medicine, for example, in which symptoms are diagnosed, and a medical treatment is administered to either subdue the symptoms or eradicate the disease. In the case of cholesterol, for example, a metaphysical approach might aim to remove perceived emotional or energetic blocks to well-being.

Because high cholesterol has been associated with various mental health conditions, some metaphysical approaches suggest that emotional or psychological imbalances may contribute to physical symptoms. Proponents of mind-body health philosophies often emphasize the importance of releasing emotional blockages, cultivating self-love, and embracing positive thinking as part of the healing journey. They may recommend practices such as affirmations, meditation, or energy work to help promote emotional well-being, which in turn is believed to support physical health.

The specific metaphysical explanation for high cholesterol involves "clogging the channels of joy." After deep inner dialogue and self-reflection, if the concept of your channels of joy being blocked resonates with you, you could ask yourself if there are reasons for the channels of joy being blocked or avenues that lead to joy in your life. Are you so engaged in responsibilities that you believe joy is frivolous, or that you "can't afford" or "don't deserve" joy? Perhaps you believe that being joyful itself is wrong because there is so much negativity around. If you seek optimal health, these ideas are worth exploring.

Even if you're not onboard with the concept of "channels of joy," the happier you are, the healthier you'll be, so seeking and accepting joy should be a goal in your life, just as much as eating well and exercising should be. Looking for healthy ways to feel joy and affirming that you welcome joy in your life are great places to start. If you have difficulty with this concept, you can seek spiritual leaders and/or mental health professionals to help you move beyond limiting beliefs.

In Hindu and Buddhist philosophies, high cholesterol is associated with imbalances in specific chakras, which then need to be balanced. High cholesterol levels may be associated with blockages in the heart chakra (associated with love and self-worth) or the solar plexus chakra (associated with power and control). Practitioners work to help improve those chakras in order to affect their patients' health.

Many people find metaphysical approaches empowering and helpful in reducing stress or improving their mindset, but it's important to note that there is limited scientific evidence directly linking specific emotional states or affirmations to changes in cholesterol levels. The mind-body connection is real and well-recognized in areas like stress and cardiovascular health, however, so the idea that emotional patterns influence a person's physical state is a reasonable assumption.

TIP

These practices may be best seen as complementary tools — helpful for supporting overall well-being, but not a replacement for medical treatment or evidence-based lifestyle interventions.

It may seem odd to discuss so many different types of therapies when there are pharmaceuticals that can reduce cholesterol levels. Everyone is different, however, and there are a wide range of conventional and complementary therapies that can work for you. It's up to you and your medical team to decide which ones are most appropriate for your lifestyle. Never has it been easier to find both conventional and complementary therapies to help people achieve their health goals.

5
Heading into the Kitchen

IN THIS PART . . .

Discover how to cook and eat to manage cholesterol.

Develop a meal plan that works for you.

Choose the right foods.

Learn the importance of extra-virgin olive oil and flavor enhancers.

Understand how to eat out with pleasure and health.

Build a pantry to save time and money.

Make a cooking schedule that works for you.

Try a seven-day meal plan to manage cholesterol.

Chapter **13**

Cooking and Eating to Manage Cholesterol

RECIPES IN THIS CHAPTER

🍳 **Tomato Basil Sauce**

🍳 **Homemade Vegetable Stock**

Homemade Chicken Stock

🍳 **Dried Beans**

🍳 **Dried Chickpeas**

🍳 **Cannellini Beans**

🍳 **Lentils**

🍳 **Baby Artichokes**

🍳 **Za'atar Spiced Pita Chips**

🍳 **Roasted Red Peppers**

🍳 **Fresh Breadcrumbs**

When people (including many medical professionals) talk about being on a meal plan to manage cholesterol, they often list major food groups that they're omitting from their diet. Flavor and incorporating ingredients that can help manage cholesterol and improve overall health usually aren't part of the discussion.

In this chapter, we show you how to cook and eat delicious foods that are packed with the nutrients you need to lessen the effects of oxidative stress and increase good cholesterol, while enjoying yourself in the process.

Cooking to Manage Cholesterol

By learning to harness the power of antioxidant-rich and high-fiber foods, along with the anti-inflammatory compounds in extra-virgin olive oil and "secret" flavor enhancers, you can eat very well while managing cholesterol. With these tips under your belt, you won't have to cut out all dairy, wheat, or meat forever. Instead, you'll learn how to plan meals using the foods that are most beneficial to your body in creative ways that are just as pleasing to the palate as they are good for you.

Planning meals

Understanding and embracing the importance of meal planning is one of the most important factors in achieving your eating goals. You can have a desire to eat well and perhaps even shop for or order healthful ingredients, but without a strategic plan that includes shopping, storing, prepping, cooking, and repurposing food weekly, you'll have trouble reaching your nutrition goals.

On the other hand, if you take the time to analyze your situation and any obstacles you face, you'll be able to put a plan in place that enables you to meet your health requirements while enjoying yourself in the process. You may not love to cook. Maybe you have someone else who cooks for you, and you're just interested in learning what's best for you to eat.

But cooking can be one of the greatest pleasures in life if you allow it to be. Many people discover the joys of the kitchen after "having to cook" for a diagnosis or a lifestyle change. Cooking empowers you to take charge of your health and the quality of the food you eat, and to develop personalized flavors that you wouldn't otherwise be able to experience.

TIP

Planning is your secret ingredient to success in the kitchen. Here are some ways to make meal planning work for you:

>> **Dedicate a set time during the week to plan meals for the next week.** Schedule meal planning in your calendar.

>> **Examine your upcoming week's schedule.** Find times that allow you to shop, prep, cook, and so on.

>> **Use technology to your advantage.** If you can't find time to shop, use online shopping services or sign up for community-supported agriculture (CSA) produce deliveries. Schedule reminders to shop, keep electronic grocery lists save recipes online so they're always with you, and so on.

To find a CSA near you in the United States, head to www.localharvest.org/csa.

>> **Set aside time to cook.** All it takes is a few hours per week to make the meals in the Sample Seven-Day Meal Plan in Chapter 14. *Remember:* You don't have to cook every day or at each meal. Take advantage of pockets of time in your

schedule to prep and create make-ahead meals. Make double and triple batches of recipes and freeze them, preportioned for busier days and nights when you know you won't have time to cook.

Find the time to make the Base Recipes in this chapter on a weekly, biweekly, or monthly basis (many of them can be frozen). This will help you to have sodium- and preservative-free ingredients on hand so making the recipes in Chapter 15 is a cinch.

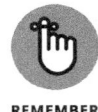

REMEMBER

Making changes is never easy. It takes time and a lot of inspiration and dedication to stay on track. The good news is that it's worth the effort. Just 30 days of eating healthful, whole foods can create positive changes in your health and happiness. Best of all, you can tailor the recipes to make them taste great and you may find a rewarding new pastime in the process.

Cooking with antioxidant-rich foods

Fruits and vegetables contain antioxidants and bioactive compounds, which are very beneficial to health. According to Mediterranean diet and lifestyle guidelines, your diet should be made up mostly of fruits and vegetables — 9 to 12 servings of fresh produce per day is the recommendation. Tasty ingredients that contain specific heart-healthy, low-density lipoprotein (LDL) cholesterol–lowering effects include apples, artichokes, blueberries, citrus fruits, cranberries, cruciferous vegetables, peas, pomegranates, raspberries, red cabbage, red grapes, red wine, strawberries, and tomatoes. Fiber-rich apples, citrus fruits, eggplants, grapes, okra, and strawberries are also readily available additions to the diet. These fruits are rich in pectin, a type of soluble fiber that lowers LDL.

REMEMBER

All fresh fruits and vegetables offer important nutrients, but if you're interested in managing cholesterol, you should be sure to include the ones we list here in your daily diets (along with others).

When managing cholesterol, healthful fats, unrefined whole-grain carbohydrates, and fiber-rich plant proteins with anti-inflammatory and antioxidant polyphenols (especially in colorful and flavorful vegetables, fruits, nuts, herbs, spices, and extra-virgin olive oil) are your greatest allies in the kitchen. A diet with the highest intake of polyphenols has been shown to be associated with a 46 percent reduced risk of cardiovascular disease.

The following ingredients are used plentifully in this book. You can use them in your own ways to help better manage cholesterol:

>> **Fresh fruits and vegetables:** Apples, artichokes, blueberries, citrus fruits, cranberries, cruciferous vegetables, okra, peas, pomegranates, raspberries,

red grapes, red wine, red cabbage, strawberries, and tomatoes are perfect choices due to their antioxidant powers and fiber content.

» **Fish:** Fish is an excellent low-fat source of protein. Salmon, tuna, and swordfish are readily available fresh and frozen and are excellent sources of not only protein, but also vitamin B6, vitamin D, niacin, selenium, and omega-3 fatty acids.

» **Whole grains:** Whole grains such as oats, barley, and 100 percent whole wheat are great sources of fiber, which can lower LDL cholesterol. These naturally fat-free grains also help you to feel full. Both barley and oats contain a specific soluble fiber called *beta-glucans* to help you manage cholesterol. Technically considered a carbohydrate, beta-glucans are especially effective at lowering LDL cholesterol levels and reducing the risk for buildup of plaque in the arteries known as *atherosclerosis.* Purchase organic whole grains whenever possible.

» **Greek yogurt:** Plain, full-fat Greek yogurt with *probiotics* (live active cultures) is known to help maintain the natural balance of organisms, known as *microbiota,* in the intestines. These beneficial bacteria may help reduce inflammation and improve gut health, which can positively impact cholesterol. Plus, the calcium content in yogurt may help block the absorption of cholesterol in the intestines.

» **Extra-virgin olive oil:** The monounsaturated fat in olive oil is called *oleic acid* and it's good for heart health. Oleic acid is the most common monounsaturated fat in the human diet. It has been shown to lower LDL cholesterol and raise high-density lipoprotein (HDL) cholesterol. Substitute good-quality extra-virgin olive oil for butter, plant seed oils, and other sources of fat in as many recipes as possible.

» **Nuts, and seeds:** Unsalted nuts are another ingredient that Americans and others on a Western diet don't take enough advantage of. Almonds can help manage cholesterol by lowering LDL cholesterol and improving HDL cholesterol; they're high in unsaturated fatty acids, fiber, phytosterols, and plant protein.

» **Beans and lentils:** Beans and lentils are rich in both soluble and insoluble fiber, which work to reduce LDL cholesterol levels. They're an important source of protein and naturally low in calories. Black beans, cannellini beans, chickpeas, kidney beans, and others can all be prepared in batches and frozen for later use. (Refer to the base recipes later in this chapter for cooking instructions.)

» **Fresh herbs and spices:** Fresh herbs and spices have known anti-inflammatory effects, which can be very beneficial for people managing cholesterol. Anti-inflammatory ingredients in general work to prevent the oxidation of LDL cholesterol, which is a key factor in the development of plaque buildup in blood vessels. Doing this reduces the risk of heart disease and other illnesses. Plus, you can incorporate them into any meal without worrying about their calories, sodium, carbohydrates, or sugar.

Avoiding unhealthful fats

If you're looking to manage your cholesterol and achieve optimal health, avoiding unhealthful fats is key. You should limit saturated fats, especially those that are found in processed and red meats and fried foods (other than those prepared in extra-virgin olive oil), because they can raise LDL cholesterol levels. Avoid trans fats from nonnatural sources altogether.

Trans fats can be found in the following:

>> Processed and packaged foods such as crackers, potato chips, and other snack foods (look for partially hydrogenated oil — or derivatives of them — on food labels)

>> Margarine

>> Shortening

>> Commercially prepared baked goods such as breads, cookies, doughnuts, and muffins

>> Nondairy creamers

>> Refrigerated commercially prepared doughs

>> Fried foods

Some places have limited the amount of trans fats in food establishments, but even in those places, it's difficult to determine who's using them and who isn't. Preparing your own food is the best way to steer clear of these unwanted additives.

THE IMPORTANCE OF EXTRA-VIRGIN OLIVE OIL

Consuming just 2 tablespoons of extra-virgin olive oil daily has been linked to a more than 40 percent reduction in the risk of heart disease and stroke. This health-promoting oil is rich in *oleic acid,* a monounsaturated fat known to support healthy cholesterol levels. However, the real strength of extra-virgin olive oil likely lies in its ability to combat

(continued)

(continued)

the harmful oxidation of LDL cholesterol — a key factor in the development of arterio-sclerotic plaques. This protective effect is largely attributed to the rare and powerful polyphenols found in high-quality extra-virgin olive oil.

To get the greatest health benefits from your olive oil, always choose one labeled "extra-virgin" and look for oils that are made with care, typically from early-harvested olives. For maximum polyphenol content, store the oil away from heat, light, and air, and enjoy it while still fresh. A peppery kick and a slight bitterness in the flavor are good signs that the oil contains a high level of these beneficial compounds.

Making Whole Foods Taste Great

Making whole foods taste as good as they are for your health is easy when you get the hang of it. By selecting the best ingredients and learning to use flavor enhancers and the proper techniques, you'll be able to coax maximum nutrition, texture, and taste out of the foods you eat.

TIP

Here are a few tricks to keep in mind:

>> **Choose local, in-season produce as much as possible.** Food that's in season and locally grown tends to have the most flavor, which means you don't have to do much with it to make it taste great.

>> **Invest in good-quality extra-virgin olive oil.** It adds flavor and nutrition to your meals, snacks, and even desserts.

>> **Consider a variety of textures.** When planning meals, make sure that you have both smooth/creamy and crisp/crunchy textures combined.

>> **Discover your favorite cooking styles.** Depending on what you're cooking, roasting, braising, and sautéing vegetables, beans, legumes, and fish usually helps to bring out the sweetness in the flavors that you're cooking them in.

>> **Use copious amounts of fresh herbs and spices.** They contain anti-inflammatory components and offer a lot of flavor. Learning to use them properly is the key to cooking healthfully without adding large amounts of salt and fat to recipes.

One thing that differentiates recipes in the United States and much of Western Europe from those found in the Mediterranean region, Latin America, Africa, and Asia is the amount of fresh herbs and spices that are used in cooking. If you're used to dining out, you've likely had even less exposure to healthy doses of these ancient flavor enhancers because fat and salt are the easiest and cheapest ways for restaurants to add flavor to food.

If you want to make your eating plan sustainable, you've got to make it taste good so you'll continue to eat that way over a long period of time. Heritage diets in the Mediterranean, Asia, Latin America, and Africa have traditionally incorporated lots of local herbs and enhanced recipes with coveted spices (some of which were local and some of which were inherited from trading).

TIP

Chapter 17 includes a recipe for an Anti-Inflammatory Spice Mix, which you can use to season vegetables, chicken, fish, beans, legumes, and any savory items that you'd like. It also describes the ritual of making an herbal tea out of dried herbs and spices.

TIP

Here are a few more ways to pack more fresh herbs and spices into your diet:

>> **Use herbs as salad greens.** A few times a week, swap out lettuce for finely chopped bunches of fresh cilantro, parsley, and mint (or your favorite herbs) and combine with diced tomatoes, cucumber, extra-virgin olive oil, and lemon juice.

>> **Season your soups and stews.** Don't be afraid to use the Anti-Inflammatory Spice Mix in Chapter 17 or your favorite mixes in your family's soup and stew recipes.

>> **Make sauces out of herbs.** Fresh pesto sauce, salsa verde, chimichurri, Moroccan chermoula, Mexican salsa, and herb chutneys are all great ways to consume more herbs.

>> **Make your own pita chips.** Use the recipe in this chapter to create your own healthy snack with nutritious *za'atar* (a Middle Eastern spice mix consisting of wild thyme, sumac, sea salt, and sesame seeds, which originally hails from Lebanon and Palestine). There are "green za'atar" mixes that exclude the sumac. *Za'atar* is also the Arabic word for wild thyme itself.

>> **Ditch the bottled dressings.** Use fresh herbs or your favorite spice along with a good-quality vinegar or lemon juice and extra-virgin olive oil to pack flavor and nutrition into your salads.

>> **Use sweet spices at breakfast.** Sprinkle cardamom, cinnamon, and ginger over Greek yogurt, oats, and cooked barley at breakfast.

>> **Make your own chai.** Blend cardamom, cinnamon, and ginger to steep with black or green tea and milk to make your own chai mixture.

>> **Rethink salt.** It's a good idea not to consume too much salt, but you do need a certain amount of sodium to function. The key is to get the right kind of sodium from the right sources. We recommend avoiding packaged and

processed foods and dining out less in order to avoid extra sodium. Prepared and packaged foods are full of sodium and make up the majority of the type of sodium that Americans consume. When you stop eating prepared and packaged foods, you can control the amount of salt you eat. Switch to unrefined sea salt, which is not expensive and can be found in organic markets and some supermarkets. Unrefined sea salt is free from chemical agents and still contains some natural trace minerals, which are beneficial to the body and help it metabolize sodium better. The recipes in this book call for unrefined sea salt.

REMEMBER

The amount of salt people like to use depends on what they're used to. You can gradually decrease the amount of salt you use, including in our recipes. Some herbs, such as baby dill, add a minerally salt-like flavor to foods without increasing your sodium intake.

TIP

Combining spices with good-quality extra-virgin olive oil helps to enhance their anti-inflammatory effects, as well as their flavor.

Preparing Base Recipes

No matter what type of cuisine you're preparing, if you learn the base recipes in this section, you'll have a much easier time.

This kitchen hack is nothing new — it's one that both homemakers and professional chefs have relied upon for centuries. For people who are interested in improving their health, however, this ancient tradition has a very modern appeal. Most commercially prepared tomato sauces, salad dressings, breadcrumbs, stocks, and so on, are full of sodium and unwanted ingredients. Plus, they don't taste as good as the homemade versions.

REMEMBER

You may notice that some commercially available stocks are labelled *low-sodium,* but that term is relative to the extremely high amounts of sodium in regular canned stock and it usually hovers around the daily maximum allowance just for one serving. Making your own stock in batches, freezing it, and keeping it on hand for when you need it is cheaper and more nutritious.

🍅 Tomato Basil Sauce

PREP TIME: ABOUT 5 MIN | COOK TIME: 20 MIN | YIELD: 6 SERVINGS

INGREDIENTS

2 tablespoons (27 grams) extra-virgin olive oil

2 large garlic cloves, peeled and minced

1½ pounds (680 grams) seeded and skinned boxed or jarred tomatoes, or 2½ pounds (1,134 grams) fresh, ripe tomatoes (if in season) (see Tip)

Unrefined sea salt, to taste

Freshly ground black pepper, to taste

4 to 5 leaves of fresh basil, oregano, or parsley

Parmigiano-Reggiano or Pecorino Romano cheese, freshly grated, for garnish

DIRECTIONS

1 In a medium saucepan, heat the oil over medium heat. Add the garlic and reduce the heat to low.

2 When the garlic begins to release its aroma (before it turns color), add the tomatoes.

3 Stir and allow the mixture to come to a boil to create caramelization on the side of the pan.

4 Add the salt, pepper, and fresh herbs; stir and cover. Reduce the heat to low, and simmer until it has thickened slightly, about 10 to 20 minutes. Taste and adjust seasonings. Serve with grated cheese.

PER SERVING: *Calories 75 (From Fat 44); Fat 5g (Saturated 1g); Cholesterol 0mg; Sodium 166mg; Carbohydrate 8g (Dietary Fiber 2g); Protein 2g.*

TIP: If you're using fresh tomatoes, place them in boiling water until their skins peel (just a few minutes), strain, and allow to cool to the touch. Peel them, remove the seeds, and cut them into chunks. Then use them in place of boxed or jarred tomatoes in Step 2.

NOTE: Most Italians make large batches of this sauce so they can have one recipe on hand at all times in the refrigerator and a spare or two in the freezer. It keeps in the refrigerator for up to a week or in the freezer for a few months.

Homemade Vegetable Stock

| PREP TIME: ABOUT 5 MIN | COOK TIME: 30 MINS | YIELD: 8 SERVINGS |

INGREDIENTS

1 medium yellow onion, halved (not peeled)

1 carrot, trimmed and halved

1 stalk celery, trimmed and halved (can include leaves, if desired)

4 ounces cherry tomatoes

4 sprigs fresh basil, with stems

1 small bunch (approximately ¾ cup or 45 grams) fresh flat-leaf parsley, with stems

16 cups (3.8 liters) water

½ teaspoon (2 grams) unrefined sea salt

DIRECTIONS

1 In a large stockpot, place the onion, carrot, celery, tomatoes, basil, and parsley. Cover with the water. Bring to a boil over high heat. Reduce the heat to medium-low. Add the salt, and simmer, uncovered, for 30 minutes.

2 Drain the stock, reserving the liquid. Discard the rest. If you're not using it right away, allow to cool and then store in the refrigerator for up to 1 week or freeze it for up to 1 month.

PER SERVING: *Calories 12 (From Fat); Fat 1g (Saturated 0g); Cholesterol 0mg; Sodium 117mg; Carbohydrate 3g (Dietary Fiber 1g); Protein 0g.*

Homemade Chicken Stock

PREP TIME: ABOUT 5 MIN | COOK TIME: 40 MIN | YIELD: 8 SERVINGS

INGREDIENTS

1 medium yellow onion, halved (not peeled)

1 medium carrot, trimmed and halved

1 medium stalk celery, trimmed and halved

1¼ pounds (567 grams) chicken bones or carcass from cooked chicken

1 teaspoon whole black peppercorns

1 dried bay leaf

16 cups (3.8 liters) water

½ teaspoon (2 grams) unrefined sea salt

DIRECTIONS

1 In a large stockpot, place the onion, carrot, celery, chicken bones, peppercorns, and bay leaf. Cover with the water. Bring to a boil over high heat. Reduce the heat to medium-low.

2 Skim off the residue that forms on top of the stock, and discard. Add the salt, and simmer, uncovered, for 40 minutes.

3 Drain the stock, reserving the liquid, and discard the rest. If you're not using the stock right away, allow it to cool, and then store it in the refrigerator for a week or freezer for up to a month.

PER SERVING: *Calories 45 (From Fat); Fat 4 g (Saturated 0 g); Cholesterol 9mg; Sodium 68mg; Carbohydrate 0g (Dietary Fiber 0g); Protein 9g.*

🍅 Dried Beans

PREP TIME: 1 HR PLUS OVERNIGHT SOAKING	COOK TIME: 30 MIN	YIELD: 8 SERVINGS

INGREDIENTS

1 cup (202 grams) dried beans (any variety)

¼ teaspoon (1 gram) salt

DIRECTIONS

1 Place the beans in a medium stockpot and cover with cold water; leave to soak overnight.

2 Drain the soaked beans and place them in a medium saucepan. Add the salt, cover the beans with water, and bring to a boil, uncovered, over high heat.

3 Reduce the heat to medium-low, cover, and let cook until the beans are tender, about 25 to 50 minutes. (It may take longer depending on the size of the beans.)

4 Drain and cool. If not using right away, store in an airtight container in the refrigerator for up to 1 week.

TIP: If you're short on time, in Step 1, place the beans in a stockpot, cover with boiling water, and leave to soak for 1 hour instead.

PER SERVING: *Calories 110 (From Fat 3); Fat 0g (Saturated 0g); Cholesterol 0mg; Sodium 52mg; Carbohydrate 20g (Dietary Fiber 6g); Protein 8g.*

TIP: Add 1 teaspoon of baking soda to the cooking water to avoid digestive issues while eating beans.

☺ Dried Chickpeas

PREP TIME: 1 HR PLUS OVERNIGHT SOAKING	COOK TIME: 30 MIN	YIELD: 8 SERVINGS

INGREDIENTS

1 cup (202 grams) dried chickpeas

¼ teaspoon (1 gram) salt

DIRECTIONS

1 Place the chickpeas in a medium stockpot and cover with cold water; leave to soak overnight.

2 Drain the soaked chickpeas and place them in a medium saucepan. Add the salt, cover the beans with water, and bring to a boil, uncovered, over high heat.

3 Reduce the heat to medium-low, cover, and let cook until the beans are tender, about 25 to 30 minutes. (It may take longer depending on the size of the chickpeas.)

4 Drain and cool. If not using right away, store in an airtight container in the refrigerator for up to 1 week.

TIP: If you're short on time, in Step 1, place the beans in a stockpot, cover with boiling water, and leave to soak for 1 hour instead.

NOTE: Add 1 teaspoon of baking soda to the cooking water to avoid digestive issues while eating chickpeas.

PER SERVING: *Calories 110 (From Fat 3); Fat 0g (Saturated 0g); Cholesterol 0mg; Sodium 52mg; Carbohydrate 20g (Dietary Fiber 6g); Protein 8g.*

☙ Cannellini Beans

PREP TIME: ABOUT 5 MIN PLUS 8 HR SOAKING	COOK TIME: 40 MIN	YIELD: 8 SERVINGS

INGREDIENTS

1 cup (202 grams) dried cannellini

4 rosemary sprigs, divided

1 tablespoon (15 milliliters) extra-virgin olive oil

¼ teaspoon (1 gram) salt

DIRECTIONS

1 In a large bowl, add the beans and enough cold water to cover them by 4 inches (10 centimeters). Let them soak in a cool place or in the refrigerator for at least 8 hours or overnight.

2 Drain the beans and transfer them to a 2-quart (1.9 liters) saucepan. Pour in enough water to cover by 1 inch (2.5 centimeters) and drop in 2 rosemary sprigs. Bring the water to a boil and then lower the heat so the water is barely at a simmer. Cook, uncovered, until the beans are tender but not mushy, with just enough liquid to cover them, about 30 to 40 minutes. (If necessary, add more water, 1 tablespoon (15 milliliters) at a time, to keep the beans covered as they simmer.)

3 Remove the beans from the heat and gently stir in the olive oil, salt, and the remaining 2 rosemary sprigs. Let the beans stand to cool and absorb the cooking liquid. If you're not using them right away, store the beans in an airtight container in the refrigerator up to 1 week.

NOTE: The end result should be tender beans with a creamy consistency in just enough liquid to coat them.

PER SERVING: *Calories 99 (From Fat 17); Fat 2g (Saturated 0g); Cholesterol 0mg; Sodium 63mg; Carbohydrate 15g (Dietary Fiber 4g); Protein 6g.*

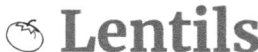 # Lentils

PREP TIME: ABOUT 5 MIN	COOK TIME: 30 MIN	YIELD: 6 SERVINGS

INGREDIENTS

1 cup (192 grams) dried lentils (any variety)

¼ teaspoon (1 gram) salt

¼ teaspoon (1 gram) freshly ground black pepper

1 bay leaf

DIRECTIONS

1 Rinse the lentils in a colander.

2 Place the lentils in a medium saucepan and add enough water to cover them twice (you should have twice as much water as lentils). Add the salt, pepper, and bay leaf.

3 Bring to a boil over high heat. Reduce the heat to low, and simmer, uncovered, until the lentils are tender, about 5 to 30 minutes, depending on the variety of lentil.

4 If you're not using them right away, store the cooked lentils in an airtight container in the refrigerator up to 1 week.

PER SERVING: *Calories 113 (From Fat 3); Fat 0g (Saturated 0g); Cholesterol 0mg; Sodium 80mg; Carbohydrate 19g (Dietary Fiber 10g); Protein 8g.*

NOTE: Red lentils are the quickest-cooking variety, followed by green, brown, and then black.

Baby Artichokes

PREP TIME: ABOUT 15 MIN	COOK TIME: 20 MIN	YIELD: 6 SERVINGS

INGREDIENTS

12 baby artichokes

Juice of 2 lemons

¼ cup (54 grams) extra-virgin olive oil

DIRECTIONS

1 Soak artichokes in warm water to clean. Drain and repeat until the water in the bowl is clear. Peel away the outside leaves of the bottom half of the artichokes. Then cut off the top quarter of the artichokes.

2 If tough, dark green leaves remain, peel those as well. (At this point, the artichoke should look like a flower, and the tough, dark leaves should all be removed, leaving only lighter-colored, more tender leaves.)

3 Add the juice of the lemons to a bowl full of cold water. Add the artichokes to prevent discoloration.

4 Bring a large pot of water to a boil over high heat. Remove the artichokes from the bowl, discarding the lemon water, and add them to the pot. Bring the water back to a boil over high heat; then reduce the heat to medium-low and simmer the artichokes until tender, about 15 to 20 minutes. Drain the artichokes and drizzle with olive oil. Turn to coat. Set aside.

PER SERVING: *Calories 67 (From Fat 34); Fat 4g (Saturated 0g); Cholesterol 0mg; Sodium 5mg; Carbohydrate 7g (Dietary Fiber 2g); Protein 1g.*

TIP: Note that this recipe calls for baby artichokes, which are smaller, more tender, and contain less of the "furry choke" in the center. If you substitute larger artichokes, you'll need to peel away much more of the exterior and remove the furry center with a spoon before eating.

☕ Za'atar Spiced Pita Chips

PREP TIME: ABOUT 2 MIN	COOK TIME: 5 MIN	YIELD: 4 SERVINGS

INGREDIENTS

4 pieces whole-wheat pita

2 tablespoons (27 grams) extra-virgin olive oil

2 tablespoons (8 grams) za'atar spice mix (see Tip)

DIRECTIONS

1 Preheat the broiler. Cut each pita loaf into 4 equal pieces.

2 Brush the olive oil on top of each piece and sprinkle za'atar over the top. Turn to coat with more oil and za'atar.

3 Bake under the broiler for 2 minutes per side or until golden. Allow to cool to room temperature and serve.

PER SERVING: *Calories 142 (From Fat 71); Fat 8g (Saturated 1g); Cholesterol 0mg; Sodium 237mg; Carbohydrate 16g (Dietary Fiber 3g); Protein 3g.*

TIP: You can find za'atar spice mix, which is usually made of wild thyme, sea salt, coriander, and sumac, in the spice isle of your supermarket, in Mediterranean or Middle Eastern markets, or online.

VARY IT! Use your own favorite spice mix instead of this one, if desired.

Roasted Red Peppers

PREP TIME: ABOUT 5 MIN	COOK TIME: 40 MIN	YIELD: 4 SERVINGS

INGREDIENTS

4 red bell peppers (keep whole)

1 tablespoon (15 milliliters) extra-virgin olive oil

DIRECTIONS

1 Preheat the oven to 500°F (260°C).

2 On a baking sheet, place the whole bell peppers. Bake until the skins are wrinkled, and the peppers are charred, about 30 to 40 minutes, being sure to turn them each time a side is charred (approximately twice during cooking).

3 Remove from the oven and cover tightly with aluminum foil to create steam. Set aside.

4 When the peppers are cool enough to handle, after about 30 minutes, cut into quarters, peel off the skin, and remove the seeds. Add to your favorite recipe or, if not eating immediately, place the pepper pieces in a jar, cover with the olive oil for additional flavor and nutrition, seal with a lid, and refrigerate up to 2 weeks. Before using, drain the oil from the peppers; reserve the oil in the refrigerator for another use.

PER SERVING: *Calories 67 (From Fat 34); Fat 4g (Saturated 0g); Cholesterol 0mg; Sodium 5mg; Carbohydrate 7g (Dietary Fiber 2g); Protein 1g.*

NOTE: Called *pepperoni rossi arrostit* in Italian, roasted red peppers are often added to antipasto platters, pastas, soups, and sauces.

NOTE: Bell peppers are a great source of vitamin C, containing approximately three times as much vitamin C as oranges. They also contain the bioactive compound *lycopene,* which is also found in tomatoes and is shown to be active against prostate and lung cancer. Cooking in extra-virgin olive oil increases the absorption of the lycopene in the peppers.

TIP: You don't need to purchase jarred peppers when you can make them easily at home. Stock up on peepers when they're on sale. You can roast them and freeze them for use later.

Fresh Breadcrumbs

PREP TIME: ABOUT 5 MIN	COOK TIME: NONE	YIELD: 16 SERVINGS

INGREDIENTS

One 8-ounce loaf dense, day-old, country-style bread

DIRECTIONS

Cut the bread into 1-inch cubes and, working in batches, place them in a food processor, being careful not to fill it more than halfway. Pulse on and off until the crumbs are as fine as possible. If not using immediately, freeze breadcrumbs in a plastic freezer bag for up to 1 month.

PER SERVING: *Calories 41 (From Fat 2); Fat 0g (Saturated 0g); Cholesterol 0mg; Sodium 92mg; Carbohydrate 8g (Dietary Fiber 0g); Protein 2g.*

Chapter **14**

Organizing the Kitchen and Meals

O rganization is the secret ingredient of all efficient kitchens. By learning how to set yourself up for success, you'll save time and money in the kitchen and at the table, while enjoying yourself in the process. Best of all, you'll be assured that you're eating in the best way possible to support your body and health goals.

In this chapter, we show you how to organize your kitchen; stock your pantry, freezer, and fridge; schedule cooking time; and meal prep. You also find out how to make the most out of dining out so that you can eat in a way that pleases your palate and meets your body's needs at the same time.

Organizing Your Kitchen

We stress the importance of cooking as much of your food at home as possible in order to maximize your nutrient intake and ensure that you're not eating ingredients that can sabotage your cholesterol management and may not be the best options for your overall health.

When people have unorganized kitchens, or when they simply lack the basic tools and utensils needed to cook with, they have a barrier that prevents them from being able to prepare food for themselves. You don't need a fancy or large kitchen to make great meals in — just one that you feel comfortable moving around and spending some time in. If you've already got a kitchen that you love, great — you can skip ahead to the next section. If you don't, however, keep reading.

Setting yourself up for success

Think of happy times that you've spent in a kitchen. Was it when you were a child? With a loved one? When you were entertaining or being entertained? Write down the words that come to mind. It might have been the comfort of spending quality time with a relative or the freedom of experimenting with a new recipe. Maybe you were at a fun gathering and everyone gathered in the kitchen to talk. Whatever comes to mind is the same type of feeling you can achieve in your own space.

Next, you'll want to stock your kitchen with what you'll need to prepare healthful and delicious recipes. If you need to move a lot of things around or "hunt" through cupboards to find ingredients or pans, cooking will require a lot more energy than needed, and you'll probably end up opting for faster, less nutritious options. Note that setting yourself up for success doesn't need to happen overnight. If you're new to all of this, take the time that you need to go through each process. It will be well worth it in the end.

TIP

Here are a few tips that can help you organize your kitchen:

>> **Clean it out!** Go through your cupboards, shelves, refrigerator, and freezer. Discard anything outdated, that isn't good for you, or that you don't like. Clean your spaces and make room for the new.

>> **Take inventory.** Look through your selections of pots and pans (stockpot, saucepans in various sizes, skillets with lids, and so on), utensils (whisks, tongs, spatulas, large wooden spoons, graters, micro planes, potato peeler, colanders), knives (chef's knife, paring knife, serrated knife), and cooking equipment (food processors, mixers). Do you have the basics? If not, make a list of what you need to purchase and a plan to do so.

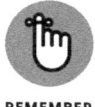

REMEMBER

You don't have to buy everything all at once or spend a fortune buying all new equipment. Wait for Black Friday sales or ask your friends and family if they have hand-me-downs. Check Facebook Marketplace or craigslist. Shop yard sales. You may be able to score some great deals!

Also, this list is just a best-case scenario. You can cook delicious and nutritious food with much less on hand!

>> **Keep things in easy reach.** Current home decorating trends have made it fashionable to keep kitchen utensils and equipment "out of sight" to make the kitchen look more like other rooms in the house. From a practicality standpoint, however, this is the worst thing to do. Have you ever walked into professional kitchens? If chefs had to keep mixers, utensils, skillets, and knives hidden away, their cooking times would increase greatly, and if you keep the items you need to cook with in cupboards, you'll be less likely to use them and discouraged when you're already tired and still need to cook. We recommend keeping what you need available and within reach. This saves time and effort.

>> **Decorate your kitchen with your own style.** Despite any limitations you may have when it comes to decorating your space, if you start out by "spicing things up" (pun intended) in the kitchen, you'll be more likely to spend time there. Think back to the question in the beginning of this section and the happy memories you've spent in the kitchen. What were the design elements that you can remember? Add photos, mementos, objects passed down by loved ones, and anything that makes your space feel special and uniquely yours. Incorporate the colors and feel that you enjoy. This will encourage you to spend more time in the space.

>> **Play music.** Make playlists of the songs that make you feel the happiest and/or peaceful. Listen to them while you're in the kitchen.

Stocking your pantry

Pantries are an ancient marvel that still have a very important role in our modern world. Those who don't understand their power often dismiss them as being necessities of the past, when people couldn't afford to do regular shopping, so they had to make meals and ingredients stretch. And although having a pantry *can* help you cut down on costs, a pantry is even more noteworthy nowadays for enabling people to quickly create healthful dishes instead of ordering unhealthful ones.

TIP

Here's a shopping list you can use to stock your pantry:

>> **Whole grains:** Old-fashioned oats, barley, millet, quinoa, farro, brown rice, amaranth, whole wheat (as well as flours made out of the same ingredients).

>> **Nuts and seeds:** Unsalted almonds, walnuts, flaxseeds, chia seeds, sesame seeds, and pumpkin seeds, as well as almond flour.

>> **Beans and legumes:** Dried chickpeas, cannellini beans, kidney beans, black beans (or your favorites), as well as red, brown, and black lentils. Because beans require soaking, it's a good idea to prepare them in advance and keep them on

hand (see Chapter 13) or keep some low-sodium canned beans on hand for when you're in a time crunch.

>> **Healthful proteins:** Jarred tuna or salmon (canned in water), and peanut or almond butter

>> **Spices and seasonings:** Keep a colorful stock of antioxidant-rich spices, good-quality extra-virgin olive oil and vinegars, and unrefined sea salt in your pantry. These are the ingredients that will boost the nutrient quotient and the flavor of your meals. See Chapters 13 and 17 for a list of individual spices and seasonings.

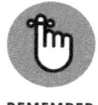

REMEMBER

Keeping good-for-you ingredients around is the foundation of a successful meal plan. A pantry saves trips to the store, allows you to save time when preparing for food, and deters you from less-healthy options.

Filling the freezer

The modern freezer is one of your best allies in your quest to eat healthfully. By keeping a well-stocked freezer, you can save time and money. Weekly grocery shopping isn't always an option and life is full of unexpected events, but when you have healthy options readily available in the freezer, you can whip up tasty, health-boosting meals in no time.

There are experts who shame the use of frozen food by saying that it's not as good as fresh. But remember, everything is relative. If having food in the freezer means that you can enjoy fish and vegetables for a fast dinner instead of ordering out or going to a restaurant, then that's the way to go. In fact, frozen vegetables and fruits retain their nutrients exceptionally well.

REMEMBER

We're not talking about ultra-processed foods — you'll want to avoid those. Instead, focus on fruits and vegetables that are frozen at their peak ripeness, which preserves their nutritional content along with seafood and lean proteins.

TIP

Here's a list of what to keep on hand in your freezer (avoid those with added sugar, salt, sauces, or other ingredients):

>> Raspberries, blueberries, and strawberries

>> Edamame

>> Carrots, green beans, artichoke hearts, peas, broccoli

>> Lean protein (whitefish, salmon, chicken breast, tofu)

>> Portions of double batches of precooked food that can be thawed in the refrigerator overnight and reheated for a second or third fast meal

Combined with pantry staples like spices, whole grains, and extra-virgin olive oil, having a freezer full of options is a great way to stay on track with your eating plan.

Focusing on the fridge

Just like the pantry and the freezer, a well-stocked refrigerator ensures that you have the best fresh ingredients on hand. You can also use your refrigerator to store pre-prepped fruits and vegetables as well as preportioned snacks and meals on the go. By planning ahead, you'll be sure to always have healthy options within reach.

TIP

Here are some foods to keep in the fridge:

>> Preportioned healthy snacks

>> Prepped (washed, dried, and cut) vegetables, fruits, and herbs to enjoy during the week

>> Fresh fruit (apples, berries, citrus, pomegranates, tomatoes)

>> Fresh vegetables (red cabbage, greens, fresh herbs, spinach, broccoli, cauliflower, onions, celery, carrots, garlic, cabbage, peppers, potatoes)

>> Dairy (plain-full fat Greek yogurt, whole milk or unsweetened almond or rice milk, fresh goat's cheese and/or aged sheep's milk cheese)

To make the most out of your groceries, pay attention to which ones "go bad" the quickest (berries, tomatoes, tomatoes, fresh herbs, spinach, and so on), and use those first. Other ingredients such as apples, citrus, pomegranates, cauliflower, onions, celery, carrots, garlic, cabbage, peppers, and tomatoes usually last longer in the refrigerator, so you can use those second.

REMEMBER

Be sure to check the use-by dates when buying dairy, and plan accordingly.

Finding Time to Cook

Time is cited as people's biggest obstacle in cooking and meal prep, and we genuinely believe that for many people that is the largest *perceived* deterrent. The reason that we use the word *perceived* is because, in actuality, time is not the thing that prevents people from cooking in the kitchen nowadays. Instead, it's the widespread devaluing of home-cooked meals.

Ever since industrialization took place from the late 18th century to the early 20th century in the United States, for example, nationwide promotional campaigns were used to convince people that cooking was a waste of time. By buying the "intelligent, modern" commercially prepared alternatives to home cooking, the consumer was believed to be cleverly saving time, which they could then use on "more important tasks." This sentiment was especially strong in post–World War II America, when women were used to working outside the home and manufacturers needed a larger demographic. The messaging used in their advertisements denounced traditional cooking as a thing of the past that could only be valued by those who weren't savvy.

Sophisticated, modern women were guided to use boxed cake mixes instead of baking from scratch, purchase bread from the grocery store instead of making it or going to an artisan bakery, buy TV dinners for the newly invented TVs, use canned vegetables and meats instead of fresh because their time was too valuable to "waste" in the kitchen. Although this story was set in America, other industrialized nations experienced their own version. Some "developing" countries are still being subject to this type of propaganda, and it has a devastating effect on health.

Fast-forward to present day, just 75 years later, and the United States, along with many places in the world, are facing epidemics like wide-spread diabetes, cholesterol and heart-related problems, and obesity. In addition, many neurodegenerative, cognitive, allergic, and developmental problems that face the modern world are a result of not eating properly and maintaining a healthful lifestyle, as well as the additives put into ultra-processed foods.

Nowadays people say that they don't have time to cook, but they can easily spend 15 to 20 minutes at a fast-food drive-through, waiting in line at a restaurant, or trying to place a food-delivery order on an app. Most times, the food that they eat after waiting that time isn't as good for them as something they could've prepared on their own. When you realize the value that healthful home cooking can provide — better health, happiness, and prevention of illness — you'll see that it's probably one of the most important things, if not the very most important thing, that you can do for yourself or others in the day.

Reclaiming your right to cook, to good food, and to taking care of yourself can be empowering. Cooking is a task that can be turned into a pleasurable pastime if you allow yourself to think of it as such. Even if you're committed to never enjoying your time in the kitchen, spending that same 15 to 20 minutes assembling a few nutritious ingredients each day will put you on the right track to optimal health.

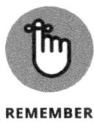

REMEMBER

Preparing and cooking from scratch healthy plant-predominant meals has been shown to be much less expensive and wasteful than buying "ready meals" — takeaway foods and ingredients without meal planning. There will be some more costly items like extra-virgin olive oil, fish, and good-quality meat, but this will be offset by the plentiful and inexpensive whole grains, beans, and vegetables.

Planning Meals

Breakfast, lunch, dinner, and snack times give you several opportunities per day to eat foods that are good for you and that you enjoy. You don't need to be a chef or a nutritionist to plan healthful meals. With the recipes in this book, and the meal planner in this section as a guide, you'll be well on your way.

TIP

Here are some suggestions to keep in mind:

>> **Make a list of what you should be eating to manage your cholesterol.** Chapters 13 and 17 list the ingredients that are best for you. Go through the list and eliminate the ones you really don't like. Then make a list of the ingredients that you enjoy and can eat. This list will become the base from which you plan your meals.

>> **To come up with complete meal formulas on your own, follow a formula.** Choose one healthy carbohydrate (whole grain or starchy vegetables), one lean protein (chicken, fish, edamame, tofu, beans, lentils), and one healthful fat (extra-virgin olive oil, avocado, nuts, or seeds). We like to add in generous doses of fresh herbs and spices for flavor and for their therapeutic properties.

>> **Know your portion sizes.** Speak with your nutrition professional or doctor to decide the amount of each food that is appropriate for your size and weight, and be sure that the correct amount of the ingredients mentioned here are what your meals consist of.

>> **Make weekly menus.** Set aside a time each week to make menus, and then grocery lists for the following week. Keep in mind what your schedule will be like — snacks needed, and so on. Do you need to prep in advance for dinner? Have breakfast and/or lunch ready to go?

>> **Create double batches of recipes whenever possible to get more bang for your buck in the kitchen.** Leftover portions can be stored in the refrigerator or frozen for enjoying later.

If you're new to the kitchen, or new to eating with cholesterol in mind, these steps may be overwhelming to you. Just start with one at a time. Each week, add a different step. In a few months' time, you'll have formed a new habit of healthy meal planning.

In the following sections, we help you set a schedule and show you a sample seven-day meal plan.

Setting a schedule that works for you

Food prep means different things for different people. If you have a traditional weekday work schedule, for example, you could set aside a few hours to a half of a day on the weekends to prep food. Or, if you have a day or two off during the week, one of those days may be your ideal time to either prep all the week's meals in advance, or at least get a head start on prepping the produce and organizing what you'd like to make and when. If you work evenings or nights, one of the mornings or afternoons of the week may be best for you. It doesn't even have to be consistent to be effective — just remember to set aside time each week to schedule meal prep into the upcoming week's schedule.

REMEMBER

If you're not used to cooking and making recipes from scratch, this step will be especially important for you. If you wait until you get home at night to decide what's for dinner, you'll be much more likely to make an unhealthy choice.

TIP

Here are some suggestions for scheduling your meal prep:

>> **Take it a week at a time.** Decide what you'd like to prepare for each meal or snack of the following week at least a few days in advance.

>> **Write it down.** Make a grocery list and schedule time in your calendar to either go shopping for the ingredients you'll need or order them.

>> **Schedule prep time.** Designate at least an hour each week (preferably the day that you get groceries or the next) to clean and trim vegetables and fruit, soak beans, and make the base recipes in Chapter 13 to have on hand for easy and efficient cooking times.

>> **Decide when to cook.** If cooking daily doesn't appeal to you or fit into your schedule, pick one or two times per week when you can cook in larger batches. If you've done the prep work, just a two-hour window will be enough time for you to cook lean proteins, beans or legumes, and complex carbohydrates that can be enjoyed throughout the week.

>> **Take advantage of your freezer.** Whenever possible, make double or triple portions of the recipes from Chapter 15 or your own good-for-you favorites that can be frozen. That way, when you know you have a busy day ahead of you where you won't be able to cook, you can thaw the premade meals in the refrigerator the night before to reheat when you get home from work the next day.

By gradually integrating these steps into your schedule, you can be assured that you'll always be a step ahead of cooking. Scheduling meals may seem unappealing at first, but you'll be delighted when you find out how simple it is to have food that nourishes your mind, body, and spirit within reach.

Looking at a sample seven-day meal plan

Using the recipes (Chapter 15) and base recipes (Chapter 13) in this book, you can create a weekly meal plan that incorporates a wide range of satisfying tastes and textures while ensuring that you're consuming a fiber- and polyphenol-rich diet that's perfect for managing cholesterol. Keep in mind that this is just a guideline — you can discuss specific quantities that are appropriate for your size, weight, and lifestyle with your nutrition professional.

Note that some of the items call for double batches so you can bring them for lunch the following day. If you're short on time, you can follow this method daily to cut down on cooking time. You can also repurpose any leftovers into soups, stews, bowls, or salads. Adding in additional portions of cooked and raw greens dressed with good-quality extra-virgin olive oil and lemon or vinegar is another great addition to the daily meals. The recipes in **bold** are included in Chapter 15 for your reference, but if you'd prefer to add in some of the ingredients listed here to your own recipes, that would work, too.

Breakfasts include black coffee or espresso, which are beloved by many, or herbal, black, and green tea, which have antioxidant benefits. For dinner, a glass of red wine, if you drink, can provide additional polyphenols to your diet, but it isn't a necessary addition.

Snacks are listed for planning purposes — you can mix them up however you choose. On a day when you aren't otherwise eating beans or legumes, hummus and *crudités* (celery sticks, carrot sticks, cherry tomatoes, broccoli and cauliflower flowerets, and so on) make a great snack. It's not important that you stick to these exact recipes, but that you follow the general principles of the meal plan in order to become familiar with the foods that will be best for you.

Day 1

Breakfast

Greek Yogurt with Honey, Pomegranate, and Avocado Parfait

Black coffee; espresso; or herbal, black, or green tea

Water

Red Cabbage, Citrus, and Carrot Slaw with Cilantro Vinaigrette (add leftover chicken, fish, or tofu for protein)

1 piece 100 percent whole-grain bread

Water

Snack

Handful of almonds

1 apple

Water

Dinner

Marinated Salmon and Brussels Sprouts over Citrus Cream Sauce

Mixed green salad dressed with extra-virgin olive oil and lemon juice or vinegar

Water

Snack

1 serving of 85 percent dark chocolate

5 walnuts

Day 2

Breakfast

Apple Cinnamon Oatmeal with Toasted Almonds

Black coffee; espresso; or herbal, black, or green tea

Glass of water

Lunch

Vegetable Stir-Fry with Edamame and Brown Rice Noodles

1 cup fresh berries

Water

Snack

½ cup plain, full-fat Greek yogurt

Water

Dinner

Italian Pasta with Creamy Lentils and Pecorino Cheese

Mixed green salad dressed with citrus juice and extra-virgin olive oil

Water

Snack

1 orange

5 almonds

Water

Day 3

Breakfast

Red Berry, Dark Chocolate, and Chia Seed Overnight Pudding

Black coffee; espresso; or herbal, black, or green tea

Water

Lunch

Avocado, Citrus, and Spinach Salad with Walnuts and White Balsamic Vinaigrette (add hard-boiled egg, grilled chicken, fish, or edamame)

Water

Snack

1 serving unsweetened Greek yogurt with a handful of blueberries

Water

Dinner

Greek Roasted "Plaki"–Style Fish with Vegetables and Brown Rice Pilaf
(make a double portion so you have leftovers for lunch tomorrow)

Water

Snack

¼ cup hummus or other bean puree with celery and carrot sticks

Water

Day 4

Breakfast

Sweet Cardamom-Scented Barley and Strawberry Pudding with Nuts

Black coffee; espresso; herbal, black, or green tea

Water

Lunch

Leftover Greek Roasted "Plaki"–Style Fish with Vegetables and Brown Rice Pilaf

Water

Snack

1 cup assorted raw vegetables (crudités) with 1 serving cottage cheese or hummus (preferably homemade)

Water

Dinner

Barley and Red Wine "Risotto" with Red Cabbage and Cannellini Beans (make a double portion for lunch tomorrow)

Green salad

Water

Snack

1 orange

10 unsalted almonds

Water

Day 5

Breakfast

Oatmeal with blueberries, flaxseeds, and almonds

Black coffee; espresso; herbal, black, or green tea

Water

Lunch

Barley and Red Wine "Risotto" with Red Cabbage and Cannellini Beans

Water

Snack

Carrot and celery sticks with tzatziki (cucumber yogurt sauce)

Water

Dinner

Spinach, Lentil, and Pomegranate Salad with grilled chicken breast or hard-boiled egg (make a double portion for lunch tomorrow)

1 piece 100 percent whole-wheat bread

Fresh Summer Berry Clafoutis

Water

Day 6

Breakfast

Cooked barley with fresh berries, honey, and toasted almonds or poached egg and avocado toast with cherry tomatoes

Black coffee; espresso; herbal, black, or green tea

Water

Lunch

Spinach, Lentil, and Pomegranate Salad with grilled chicken breast or hard-boiled egg

Water

Snack

1 apple with 1 teaspoon peanut butter

Water

Dinner

Artichoke, Pea, and Cherry Tomato Salad with Lemon and Basil Dressing

Herb-marinated chicken breast

1 piece whole-grain bread

Water

Snack

½ cup unsweetened Greek yogurt with ¼ cup chopped fresh strawberries

Water

Day 7

Breakfast

Chocolate Ginger Waffles with Vanilla Berry Syrup

Black coffee; espresso; herbal, black, or green tea

Water

Lunch

Vegetable minestrone made with homemade stocks (see Chapter 13), beans, and quinoa

1 piece whole-grain bread

Moroccan Carrot Salad

Water

Snack

¼ cup olives (rinsed if in brine and drizzled with extra-virgin olive oil and spices of your choice)

Water

Dinner

Roasted fish of your choice prepared with extra-virgin olive oil and Anti-Inflammatory Spice Mix (Chapter 17) and brown rice or barley

Red Cabbage, Citrus, and Carrot Slaw with Cilantro Vinaigrette

Italian Grape Harvest Cake with Cinnamon–Red Wine Reduction

Water

Snack

1 cup raw broccoli and/or cauliflower with 2 tablespoons hummus

Water

Eating Out with Pleasure and Health in Mind

Eating out is more common now than it has ever been in history. It's unrealistic to expect people to not eat out while they're following a specific meal plan. Other than a modern-day necessity, eating out can be one of life's greatest pleasures.

With a few simple tricks up your sleeve, you can develop dining-out habits that will help you to do so without your health suffering.

TIP

Here are a few tips to keep in mind:

>> **Know what works.** By the time you've read through this book, you'll already see some recurring trends — whole, plant-based foods, fiber, healthy fats such as avocado and extra-virgin olive oil, fresh herbs and spices, colorful vegetables, and oily fish. In the restaurant world, that may look like a large salad with grilled chicken and fish and extra-virgin olive oil/lemon juice on the side, grilled or roasted fish without the sauce and vegetables dressed with extra-virgin olive oil, vegetable- or seafood-based soups, hummus or other beans/legumes with whole-grain types of bread, and so on.

>> **Beware of the hidden.** Avoid premade sauces, condiments, and dressings, as well as processed and sugary foods.

>> **Be prepared.** Have a list of "go-to" restaurants and menu items that you can rely on to find the types of dishes that you need.

>> **Limit alcohol.** If you're drinking, opt for a single serving of polyphenol-rich red wine. Otherwise, opt for water with lemon juice or herbal or green tea.

>> **Call in advance.** If you're dining with a group and you don't want to have to ask a lot of questions in front of the group, call ahead and ask to have a special dish prepared that you can eat.

>> **Pay attention to portion sizes.** Nowadays, many restaurants serve family-size platters instead of individual portion-size plates. Ask your nutrition professional what constitutes a portion for you, and don't be afraid to share or take the excess home to enjoy for another meal.

TIP

In addition to going out to restaurants, you may be dining at a friend or family member's house. If you know that their food doesn't fit into your lifestyle plan, bring something that's shareable that you can safely eat. Try bringing one of the recipes in this book! You may find that others like it, too, and you'll have solved a problem for the future.

Chapter **15**

Recipes

RECIPES IN THIS CHAPTER

🕙 **Apple Cinnamon Oatmeal with Toasted Almonds**

🕙 **Red Berry, Dark Chocolate, and Chia Seed Overnight Pudding**

🕙 **Greek Yogurt with Honey, Pomegranate, and Avocado Parfait**

🕙 **Sweet Cardamom-Scented Barley and Strawberry Pudding with Nuts**

🕙 **Chocolate Ginger Waffles with Vanilla Berry Syrup**

🕙 **Pomegranate and Walnut Dip with Za'atar Spiced Pita Chips**

🕙 **Spiced Quinoa and Lentil Sliders**

🕙 **Italian Barley, Bean, and Mixed Vegetable Soup**

🕙 **Red Lentil "Meatballs" with Tomato Basil Sauce**

I n the United States alone, according to Cleveland Clinic, one in three adults has high cholesterol and for more than half of them, treatment isn't helping enough or they're not being treated in the first place. A cholesterol-friendly meal plan is a great way to prevent cholesterol from being raised and protect against the effects of oxidative stress (see Chapter 4).

For years, people were told that all they needed to do to make a food or recipe cholesterol-friendly was to make sure that it was low in fat. Nowadays, however, we have a completely different and comprehensive approach to designing cholesterol-friendly meals. This highly effective and flavor-forward approach combines anti-inflammatory foods with high fiber and healthy fats. Adopting this approach to eating means that you can not only lower your total cholesterol but also, more important, prevent the illnesses that are associated with having high cholesterol.

Long gone are the days when eating cholesterol-friendly foods meant giving up tasty and familiar flavors. The easy and mouth-watering recipes in this chapter focus not only on important ingredients that reduce "bad" cholesterol (like fiber, whole grains, and healthy fats), but also on the delicious bioactive compounds in colorful plants, which add flavor, decrease the oxidation of cholesterol, and reduce inflammation.

🍳 Classic Hummus with Crudités

Herb-Roasted "Plaki"-Style Fish with Vegetables and Brown Rice Pilaf

Marinated Salmon and Brussels Sprouts over Citrus Cream Sauce

🍳 Vegetable Stir-Fry with Edamame and Brown Rice Noodles

🍳 Barley and Red Wine "Risotto" with Red Cabbage and Cannellini Beans

🍳 Italian Pasta with Creamy Lentils and Pecorino Cheese

🍳 Red Cabbage, Citrus, and Carrot Slaw with Cilantro Vinaigrette

🍳 Artichoke, Pea, and Cherry Tomato Salad with Lemon and Basil Dressing

🍳 Spinach, Lentil, and Pomegranate Salad

🍳 Moroccan Carrot Salad

🍳 Avocado, Citrus, and Spinach Salad with Walnuts and White Balsamic Vinaigrette

🍳 Individual Spiced Apple Pies with Almond and Oatmeal Crust

🍳 Italian Grape Harvest Cake with Cinnamon–Red Wine Reduction

🍳 Decadent Dark Chocolate Mousse with Strawberries

🍳 Fresh Summer Berry Clafoutis

🍳 Orange and Olive Oil Walnut Cake

In this chapter, you prepare boast-worthy breakfasts, satisfying lunches and dinners, and desserts that will dazzle your guests — all while helping to keep your cholesterol in check.

Finding Cholesterol-Friendly Foods

So, what exactly *are* cholesterol-friendly foods? And do you have to give up flavor to manage your cholesterol? (Spoiler: Definitely not!) As you'll see in the recipes in this chapter, cholesterol-friendly foods:

>> **Reduce inflammation.** Controlling inflammation is key to cholesterol management (see Chapter 6). Because inflammation contributes to *atherosclerosis* (plaque buildup in the arteries) and increases the risk of heart complications, choosing an anti-inflammatory diet can set you up for success with cholesterol management. Anti-inflammatory ingredients include apples, artichokes, black pepper, blueberries, chili pepper, cinnamon, citrus fruits (including grapefruits, lemons, and oranges), cranberries, cruciferous vegetables (think arugula, broccoli, and kale), dark chocolate, fatty fish (such as herring, mackerel, and salmon), garlic, ginger, onions, peas, pomegranates, raspberries, red cabbage, red grapes, red wine, strawberries, tomatoes, turmeric, and a variety of herbs.

Polyphenols are a class of chemical compounds found in plants that act as antioxidants and have anti-inflammatory properties. Foods high in polyphenols include extra-virgin olive oil, fresh fruits and vegetables, herbs and spices, chamomile and green teas, and seeds.

And don't t underestimate the antioxidant and anti-inflammatory properties of good-quality extra-virgin olive oil — we love olive oil so much that we wrote an entire book about it: *Olive Oil For Dummies* (published by John Wiley & Sons).

>> **Include healthful fats.** Healthful fats, which include monounsaturated and polyunsaturated fats, not only add flavor and substance to your meals but also help to lower cholesterol. That's a win-win! They include extra-virgin olive oil (we won't stop preaching about it!), nuts, seeds, and fish. These ingredients all play a major role in the recipes in this chapter.

>> **Are high in fiber.** Fiber has long been touted as having the ability to lower low-density lipoprotein (LDL) cholesterol. For this reason, our recipes include whole grains (like barley, oatmeal, and whole wheat), as well as beans and lentils. Bonus: These naturally fat-free ingredients also help you to feel full. Beans and lentils can help you to burn fat and build muscle as well!

We combined the list of anti-inflammatory foods with the foods that are full of healthful fats and those that are high in fiber and came up with recipes to help you enjoy your meals with both health *and* pleasure in mind.

TIP

Plenty of foods are anti-inflammatory *and* high in fiber or anti-inflammatory *and* a good source of healthful fats. For example, extra-virgin olive oil is a healthful fat that is also anti-inflammatory, and many of the fruits and vegetables that reduce inflammation are also high in fiber. You don't have to work too hard to find foods that pull double duty.

CHOOSING EXTRA-VIRGIN OLIVE OIL

A good quality extra-virgin olive oil — a key ingredient in the Mediterranean diet — will help you add flavor and healthful fats to your diet. It will also provide you with the polyphenols needed to help combat inflammation. Swapping extra-virgin olive oil for unhealthful fats is a great way to manage cholesterol. We love olive oil so much, that we wrote *Olive Oil For Dummies*, which takes a deep dive into why this single ingredient is so important.

Here are some tips for choosing a good-quality olive oil:

- **Always look for *extra-virgin*.** This ensures that the product meets certain standards and will have a lower acidity rate than plain, "virgin" olive oils.

- **Look for the harvest date or "best by" date.** Usually, extra-virgin olive oil contains the most bioactive compounds, which help combat inflammation within a year of harvest. Most bottles of extra-virgin olive oil are stamped with a "best by" date that is two years after harvest, so try to use it a year before that.

(continued)

(continued)

- **Look for health claims on the label.** If a bottle has claims on it — such as *low acidity, high polyphenol,* or a heart health claim — that's a good thing. Refer to the brand's website to learn more.

- **Look for quality seals.** Quality seals such as Protected Origin Designation or those from the North American Olive Oil Association ensure quality.

- **Look for single-estate extra-virgin olive oil.** You can visit the estate's website to see where the product came from, how it was treated, and what standards the estate is known for,

Amy Riolo Selections Extra-Virgin Olive Oil (www.amyriolo.com/store-1/p/extravergin-olive-oil) is an extra-virgin olive oil made exclusively from Carolea olives with a low acidity and high level of polyphenol content. It was also given the Slow Food Presidium that protects small scale food production based on traditional practices at risk of extinction.

Simon Poole's Positively Good For You Heart-Healthy Extra-Virgin Olive Oil (www.pgfy.com) is available in the United Kingdom. Made from 100 percent Picual olives, it contains a minimum of 300 milligrams per kilogram, which is at least twice the level seen in most extra-virgin olive oils and provides a wonderful synergy of taste and health benefits, promoting a healthy heart.

Both of these extra-virgin olive oils work well with the recipes in this book and can enhance the flavor and nutrient content at any time of day.

Breakfast

There are many different and highly personal theories about what breakfast should be like, when it should be eaten, how it should be eaten, and if it should be eaten at all. In some cultures, people prefer short and sweet breakfasts first thing in the morning to get them fueled up for their days. In other cultures, people prefer protein-rich breakfasts that keep them feeling full until dinnertime.

In Italy, there is a saying *"Colazione da re, pranzo da principe, e cena da povero,"* which translates to "Breakfast like a king, lunch like a prince, and dinner like a pauper." This cultural attitude implies that the first meal of the day should be the largest and most caloric — a practice that was especially important for people who worked in the fields and needed a large meal in the morning to help sustain them through a day full of intense physical activity. Lunch was still hefty ("like a prince") because there was much work to be done, and dinner was light ("like a pauper") because the physical activity was done.

Arranging heavier meals around a time when you get more activity and lighter meals around times that you don't, in general, is good advice no matter where you live. In the Indian Ayurvedic tradition, it's important to plan your meals in accordance with the seasons. This eating plan recommends that in winter, for example, you should eat the largest and most caloric meals when the sun is at its peak in order to achieve optimal health.

Many people who are following a certain health plan yet don't have a lot of time in the morning prefer to make breakfasts ahead or grab a quick smoothie or breakfast bar on the go. With the current popularity of *intermittent fasting* (in which people alternate between periods of eating and periods of fasting), some people skip breakfast altogether and begin eating at lunchtime. (Check with your healthcare professional before embarking on this regime to see if it's appropriate for your situation.) But even if you're eating later in the day, there's no reason not to indulge in the comforting flavors of traditional breakfasts.

Put some thought into which breakfast style, type, and time suits you and your lifestyle best. When you figure that out, you can enjoy making and eating recipes such as those in this chapter.

Apple Cinnamon Oatmeal with Toasted Almonds

PREP TIME: ABOUT 5 MIN	COOK TIME: 25 MIN	YIELD: 4 SERVINGS

INGREDIENTS

1 cup (81 grams) steel-cut oats

4 apples, washed, cored, and diced

1 teaspoon (3 grams) ground cinnamon

½ cup (73 grams) whole raw almonds, chopped and toasted

4 teaspoons (28 grams) raw honey

1 cup (100 grams) unsweetened almond milk

DIRECTIONS

1 In a medium saucepan, bring 4 cups (946 milliliters) water to a boil over high heat. Stir in the oats.

2 Reduce the heat to medium and cook for 10 minutes. Add in the apples, cinnamon, and almonds, and cook, stirring occasionally, until the oatmeal is tender, about 10 to 15 minutes.

3 Stir in the raw honey and place into 4 individual bowls. Drizzle one-quarter of the almond milk over each bowl and add more cinnamon over the top (if desired). Serve warm or allow to cool to room temperature and store in the refrigerator until serving.

PER SERVING: *Calories 307 (From Fat 103); Fat 11g (Saturated 1g); Cholesterol 0mg; Sodium 8mg; Carbohydrate 49g (Dietary Fiber 9g); Protein 7g.*

TIP: Keep cooked oatmeal (without the fruit) on hand for busy mornings. Add in berries, apples, or a diced fruit of your choice before eating.

VARY IT! Steel-cut oats offer the most nutrition, but you can substitute old-fashioned oats to save time in a pinch. Add in ¼ cup (22 grams) unsweetened cocoa powder to make chocolate oatmeal, if desired.

Red Berry, Dark Chocolate, and Chia Seed Overnight Pudding

PREP TIME: ABOUT 5 MIN PLUS CHILLING TIME	COOK TIME: NONE	YIELD: 4 SERVINGS

INGREDIENTS

½ cup (43 grams) cocoa powder

¾ teaspoon (4 grams) unrefined sea salt

1 cup (140 grams) chia seeds

¼ cup (85 grams) raw honey

2⅔ cups (267 grams) unsweetened almond milk

1 teaspoon (4 grams) vanilla extract

1 cup (123 grams) raspberries

1 cup (166 grams) sliced strawberries

½ cup (48 grams) sliced almonds,

2 ounces (58 grams) 90% dark chocolate, shaved, for garnish

DIRECTIONS

1 In a medium mixing bowl, whisk together the cocoa powder and sea salt. Mix in the chia seeds and honey. Pour in the almond milk and vanilla, and stir until combined well. Fold in the raspberries and strawberries.

2 Pour into 4 pudding dishes or small dessert bowls. Cover and refrigerate for at least 1 hour or preferably overnight.

3 Garnish each with one-quarter of the sliced almonds and shaved dark chocolate and serve.

PER SERVING: *Calories 466 (From Fat 235); Fat 26g (Saturated 6g); Cholesterol 0mg; Sodium 365mg; Carbohydrate 56g (Dietary Fiber 23g); Protein 13g.*

TIP: The longer this pudding sits, the thicker and smoother it will become.

NOTE: Both the Aztec and Mayan civilizations used cacao and chia seeds in their diets for their medicinal purposes. The use of chia seeds in this recipe act as a thickener, replacing the need for corn or potato starch while adding protein, healthful fats, iron, magnesium, phosphorous, and zinc.

VARY IT! Use soy, rice, or regular milk instead of almond milk if you prefer.

⬤ Greek Yogurt with Honey, Pomegranate, and Avocado Parfait

PREP TIME: ABOUT 10 MIN	COOK TIME: NONE	YIELD: 4 SERVINGS

INGREDIENTS

3 cups (680 grams) plain, full-fat Greek yogurt

1 cup (174 grams) pomegranate arils

2 ripe medium avocados, peeled and sliced

4 teaspoons (28 grams) raw honey

½ teaspoon (1 gram) ground cinnamon

½ teaspoon (1 gram) ground cardamom

DIRECTIONS

1 Place ¾ cup (170 grams) Greek yogurt in each of 4 bowls or dessert cups. Top each with ¼ cup (44 grams) pomegranate arils, slices of ½ avocado, and 1 teaspoon (1 gram) honey.

2 Mix together the cinnamon and cardamom. Dust each parfait with ¼ of the mixture.

3 Serve immediately or store in the refrigerator until serving.

PER SERVING: *Calories 327 (From Fat 166); Fat 18g (Saturated 6g); Cholesterol 0mg; Sodium 66mg; Carbohydrate 28g (Dietary Fiber 6g); Protein 17g.*

TIP: This delicious and nutritious breakfast can do double duty as a snack between meals or post workout.

NOTE: If you plan on refrigerating the parfaits for more than a few minutes, be sure to sprinkle the avocado slices with fresh lemon juice and turn to coat before adding to the parfait so they don't turn color.

🍅 Sweet Cardamom-Scented Barley and Strawberry Pudding with Nuts

| PREP TIME: ABOUT 10 MIN | COOK TIME: 1 HR 30 MIN | YIELD: 6 SERVINGS |

INGREDIENTS

1¼ cups (225 grams) pearl barley

2 cups (200 grams) milk or unsweetened almond milk

1 cup (166 grams) strawberry slices

2 tablespoons (42 grams) raw honey

½ cup (50 grams) plain walnuts, chopped

1 teaspoon (1 gram) ground cardamom

DIRECTIONS

1 Bring a large saucepan three-quarters full of water to a boil over high heat. Add the barley and cook until tender, about 20 to 30 minutes.

2 In a medium saucepan, combine the cooked barley with the milk and stir. Cover and cook the mixture over high heat just until it comes to a boil. Reduce the heat to medium-low and cook, stirring occasionally, until thickened, about 20 minutes, or according to package directions.

3 Stir in the strawberries, honey, and most of the walnuts. Spoon the pudding in small dessert bowls and garnish with the remaining walnuts and cardamom.

PER SERVING: *Calories 241 (From Fat 62); Fat 7g (Saturated 1g); Cholesterol 0mg; Sodium 4mg; Carbohydrate 42g (Dietary Fiber 8g); Protein 6g.*

NOTE: Barley is rich in fiber, especially beta-glucan, which may reduce cholesterol and blood sugar levels.

TIP: You can make large batches of barley and keep it in the refrigerator to add to soups and salads and use as a rice alternative when needed.

VARY IT! Use brown rice or wheat berries instead of barley, if desired. Use pomegranate or your favorite fruit instead of strawberries.

⟳ Chocolate Ginger Waffles with Vanilla Berry Syrup

PREP TIME: ABOUT 5 MIN	COOK TIME: 10 MIN	YIELD: 4 SERVINGS

INGREDIENTS

2 large eggs

2 teaspoons (8 grams) vanilla extract, divided

½ cup (50 grams) milk or unsweetened almond milk

2 tablespoons (14 grams) flaxseeds

2 cups (240 grams) barley flour or whole-wheat flour

¼ cup (22 grams) unsweetened cocoa powder

1 teaspoon (1 gram) ground ginger

1 teaspoon (1 gram) baking soda

2 cups (300 grams) mixed berries (blueberries, raspberries, strawberries, and so on)

⅓ cup (112 grams) raw honey, melted

2 teaspoons (10 grams) unsalted butter, melted, or oil, for waffle maker

DIRECTIONS

1 Preheat the waffle maker.

2 In a medium bowl, whisk together the eggs, 1 teaspoon (4 grams) of the vanilla, and the milk.

3 Stir in the flaxseeds, flour, cocoa, ginger, and baking soda, mixing well to combine. If the batter seems too thick, add water, 1 tablespoon (15 milliliters) at a time to make a batter the consistency of a slightly thicker-than-normal pancake batter. Set aside.

4 In a medium bowl, combine the berries with the remaining 1 teaspoon (4 grams) of vanilla and stir in the honey.

5 Brush the waffle maker with the melted butter or oil. Pour approximately ⅓ cup (79 milliliters) of batter onto the hot waffle maker. Using a spoon, spread the batter to the corners before shutting the lid. Cook until the waffles are puffy and cooked through, about 3 to 5 minutes. Be careful not to over-cook. Spoon the berry mixture over the warm waffles, and serve immediately.

PER SERVING: *Calories 283 (From Fat 50); Fat 6g (Saturated 2g); Cholesterol 74mg; Sodium 28mg; Carbohydrate 55g (Dietary Fiber 8g); Protein 9g.*

VARY IT! For regular whole-grain waffles, remove the chocolate and the ginger. Add your spices of choice, such as cinnamon, and follow the recipe the same way.

Savory Appetizers and Small Plates

Savory appetizers and small plates are among many chefs' favorite dishes to create. This is because they allow for creativity and variation. With these recipes, you can experiment and create the excitement that leads to a delicious and memorable meal. In fact, when dining out, many people prefer to make their meals out of several appetizers and small plates, allowing them to nibble on various flavor combinations instead of choosing a main dish.

The recipes in this section are meant to be shared prior to a traditional meal or enjoyed alone alongside a green salad or other cruciferous vegetables for lunch or dinner. They can also do double duty as nutritious and tasty snacks when needed.

TIP

Having a party? Try serving these dips, croquettes, and salads on a buffet. Guests will be so impressed by their appearance and depth of flavor that they won't even realize they were created as a part of a cholesterol-friendly diet. Their global appeal will be appreciated by people of all ages, including vegetarians, vegans, and those following a gluten-free diet.

When developing these recipes, we intentionally chose ingredients that are known to be beneficial in lowering LDL cholesterol, reducing oxidative stress, and increasing high-density lipoprotein (HDL, or "good") cholesterol. We also incorporate powerful bioactive compounds and include nuts, legumes, and seeds — all ingredients that people following "modern" diets tend to leave out.

Heritage diets (specific food patterns rooted in a culture's traditional cuisine) such as the Mediterranean diet recommend eating one serving of nuts, seeds, beans, and/or legumes daily. They also recommend basing meals on the same plant-based ingredients we highlight in this section and dressing them all with good-quality extra-virgin olive oil. Our goal is to help you enjoy a wide range of flavors and nutrients while increasing your intake of fiber and antioxidants and your overall fullness. With these dishes, you'll be sure to get your recommended intake of fiber, as well as other vitamins and minerals, while enjoying yourself in the process!

🍅 Pomegranate and Walnut Dip with Za'atar Spiced Pita Chips

PREP TIME: ABOUT 5 MIN	COOK TIME: NONE	YIELD: 4 SERVINGS

INGREDIENTS

1 recipe Roasted Red Peppers (see Chapter 13)

⅓ cup (36 grams) fresh plain breadcrumbs (see Chapter 13)

⅓ cup (33 grams) walnuts, divided

4 cloves garlic, sliced

Juice of 1 lemon

4 tablespoons (80 grams) pomegranate molasses, divided

Pinch of cayenne pepper or paprika

¼ cup (54 grams) extra-virgin olive oil

Pinch unrefined sea salt, to taste, if necessary

Za'atar Spiced Pita Chips (see Chapter 13), to serve

DIRECTIONS

1 In a food processor, combine the peppers, the breadcrumbs, the walnuts (reserving 1 walnut for garnish), the garlic, the lemon juice, 3 tablespoons (60 grams) of the pomegranate molasses, and the cayenne pepper. Pulse on and off, gradually pouring in the olive oil with the food processor running until a smooth paste (the consistency of hummus) is formed. If the consistency is too thin, add more breadcrumbs; if it's too thick, add more lemon juice. Taste and adjust salt and cayenne, if desired.

2 Spoon the mixture onto a plate. Use the back of a large spoon to make a well in the center of the puree. Drizzle with the remaining 1 tablespoon (20 grams) pomegranate molasses. Place the remaining walnut in the center and serve immediately, or refrigerate, covered, until serving at room temperature with Za'atar Spiced Pita Chips.

PER SERVING: *Calories 480 (From Fat 279); Fat 31g (Saturated 4g); Cholesterol 0mg; Sodium 308mg; Carbohydrate 47g (Dietary Fiber 6g); Protein 7g.*

TIP: Use the recipe in Chapter 13 to make your own roasted red peppers, or substitute the rinsed jarred variety from the store if necessary. Use the recipe in Chapter 13 to make your own sodium- and preservative-free fresh breadcrumbs, or buy them at the store if you're short on time. You can find pomegranate molasses online or at Middle Eastern stores, or you can make your own: Cook down 1 cup (250 grams) of unsweetened pomegranate juice until it becomes very thick and add 1 teaspoon (4 grams) of sugar.

NOTE: This recipe is a traditional Arabic dish called *muhammara*, which means "to make red" in Arabic. It's a delicious snack or appetizer on its own, and it pairs well with chicken and turkey meat.

VARY IT! Dress up leftover chicken and turkey with a smear of this delicious dip.

⊙ Spiced Quinoa and Lentil Sliders

PREP TIME: ABOUT 10 MIN	COOK TIME: 10 MIN	YIELD: 4 SERVINGS

INGREDIENTS

1 cup (198 grams) Lentils (see Chapter 13)

1 cup (185 grams) cooked quinoa

¼ cup (56 grams) full-fat plain Greek yogurt

1 bunch fresh parsley leaves, washed, dried, and finely chopped, divided

1 Roasted Red Pepper (see Chapter 13), finely diced

1 teaspoon (1 gram) smoked paprika

½ teaspoon (2 grams) unrefined sea salt

¼ teaspoon (1 gram) freshly ground black pepper

2 tablespoons (27 grams) extra-virgin olive oil

8 large lettuce leaves (Bibb, Boston, or Romaine)

4 ounces (113 grams) soft goat cheese, to serve (optional)

DIRECTIONS

1 In a food processor or small blender, puree the lentils until smooth. Spoon into a small bowl, using a spatula to scrape everything from the bottom and sides. Add the quinoa, yogurt, parsley (reserving 1 tablespoon [15 milliliters] for garnish), red pepper, paprika, salt, and pepper.

2 Using your hands or a ⅓ cup (79 milliliters) measure or your hands, shape the mixture into 8 patties. Place them onto a cutting board or dish.

3 In a large, wide skillet, heat the olive oil over medium–high heat. Coat the bottom of the pan when warm and add the patties, gently pressing down on each one and flattening to approximately ½ inch. Cook until browned, about 3 to 4 minutes per side.

4 Arrange the lettuce leaves on the bottom of a serving platter. Top with the patties. Top each patty with a piece of goat cheese. Sprinkle with the remaining 1 tablespoon (15 milliliters) of parsley and serve. To eat, wrap the excess lettuce around the burger, like a "keto burger."

PER SERVING: *Calories 203 (From Fat 85); Fat 9g (Saturated 1g); Cholesterol 0mg; Sodium 245mg; Carbohydrate 22g (Dietary Fiber 6g); Protein 8g.*

TIP: You can make the patties in advance, store them in the refrigerator, and reheat before serving. If using as an appetizer, this dish pairs well with the Citrus-Marinated Salmon over Cucumber Yogurt Dill Sauce and the Vegetable Stir-Fry with Edamame and Brown Rice Noodles in the next section.

NOTE: You can substitute drained and rinsed red peppers for the roasted red peppers if desired.

🍅 Italian Barley, Bean, and Mixed Vegetable Soup

| PREP TIME: ABOUT 15 MIN | COOK TIME: 50 MIN | YIELD: 8 SERVINGS |

INGREDIENTS

2 tablespoons (27 grams) extra-virgin olive oil

1 stalk celery, diced

1 carrot, diced

1 large yellow onion, diced

2 cloves garlic, peeled and finely diced

2 cups (480 grams) Tomato Basil Sauce (see Chapter 13), boxed chopped tomatoes, or canned reduced-sodium diced tomatoes

4 cups (280 grams) chopped savoy cabbage

1 cup (177 grams) Cannellini Beans (see Chapter 13)

½ teaspoon (2 grams) unrefined sea salt

¼ teaspoon (1 gram) freshly ground black pepper

1 cup (157 grams) cooked barley

4 cups (1 liter) Homemade Chicken Stock or Homemade Vegetable Stock (see Chapter 13) or water

½ teaspoon (1 gram) crushed red chili flakes

DIRECTIONS

1 Add the olive oil to a large, heavy-bottomed saucepan or Dutch oven over medium heat. Add the celery, carrot, and onion.

2 Sauté until golden, approximately 4 minutes. Add the garlic, stir, and cook for another minute. Add the tomato sauce, cabbage, beans, salt, and pepper. Stir and simmer for 5 minutes.

3 Add the barley to the vegetable mixture along with the stock and the crushed red chili flakes. Bring to a boil over high heat. Reduce the heat to medium-low and simmer, covered, until the vegetables are tender, about 40 minutes. Serve hot.

PER SERVING: Calories 133 (From Fat 49); Fat 5g (Saturated 1g); Cholesterol 0mg; Sodium 150mg; Carbohydrate 19g (Dietary Fiber 5g); Protein 4g.

TIP: This soup gets better as it sits, making it the perfect cook-ahead dish. You can also freeze it in individual containers to reheat later. Serve larger portions with salad for a healthful and satisfying meal.

NOTE: These types of Italian soups are known as *minestre* and have been nourishing people since antiquity. Their appeal is every bit as satisfying now as it was then.

☙ Red Lentil "Meatballs" with Tomato Basil Sauce

PREP TIME: ABOUT 15 MIN PLUS RESTING TIME	COOK TIME: 40 MIN	YIELD: 6 SERVINGS

INGREDIENTS

1 cup (192 grams) red lentils, rinsed

2 tablespoons (27 grams) extra-virgin olive oil

1 small yellow onion, chopped

2 cups (142 grams) chopped broccoli

1 cup (30 grams) baby spinach

1 clove garlic, peeled and sliced

¼ cup (6 grams) freshly chopped basil

1 cup (108 grams) fresh plain breadcrumbs (see Chapter 13)

½ teaspoon (2 grams) unrefined sea salt

¼ teaspoon (1 gram) freshly ground black pepper

1 recipe Tomato Basil Sauce (see Chapter 13)

DIRECTIONS

1 Preheat the oven to 425°F (218°C).

2 Place 2 cups (480 milliliters) water in a medium pot and bring to boil over high heat. Add the lentils, reduce the heat to low, and cover. Allow to cook until the lentils are soft and water has evaporated, about 10 to 15 minutes. Remove from the heat and allow to cool while sautéing the vegetables.

3 In a large, wide skillet, heat the olive oil over medium heat. Add the onion and sauté until golden, about 3 to 4 minutes. Add the broccoli, turning to coat in the oil. Add ¼ cup (60 milliliters) water and allow to cook until tender, about 5 to 10 minutes. Add the spinach, turn to coat, and cook until wilted, about 1 minute. Stir in the garlic and basil and turn to coat. Remove from the heat.

4 Add the cooled lentils and the sautéed vegetables to a food processor and pulse until a uniform mixture is formed. Spoon the mixture into a bowl and add the breadcrumbs, salt, and pepper. Stir to combine. Place the bowl in the refrigerator for 15 minutes.

5 Place the tomato sauce in a large pot and bring to a boil over medium heat. Reduce the heat to low and allow to simmer.

6 Line a baking sheet with parchment paper. Remove the mixture from the refrigerator and use your hands or a small ice-cream scoop to form 2-inch (5-centimeter) meatballs. Place on the parchment and bake until golden on top and solid, about 20 minutes. To serve, place on a platter and spoon the sauce over the top.

(continued)

PER SERVING: *Calories 323 (From Fat 101); Fat 11g (Saturated 2g); Cholesterol 0mg; Sodium 315mg; Carbohydrate 45g (Dietary Fiber 7g); Protein 13g.*

TIP: If you're making these for company, you can make both the tomato sauce and the meatballs a day in advance. Heat before serving.

NOTE: The amount of breadcrumbs needed for the recipe will vary depending on the water content in the individual vegetables. Use more if the mixture is too loose to form meatballs and less if it thickens up before using the full cup.

VARY IT! Swap the broccoli for mushrooms and red lentils for brown, if desired.

Classic Hummus with Crudités

PREP TIME: ABOUT 15 MIN	COOK TIME: NONE	YIELD: 8 SERVINGS

INGREDIENTS

2 cups (400 grams) Dried Chickpeas, peeled, divided (see Chapter 13)

1 ice cube

4 tablespoons (54 grams) extra-virgin olive oil, divided

Juice of 1 lemon

1 garlic clove

2 tablespoons (30 grams) tahini sauce

Unrefined sea salt, to taste

Freshly ground black pepper, to taste

Smoked paprika, for garnish

6 celery stalks, trimmed and cut into thirds for serving

2 cups (298 grams) cherry tomatoes, for serving

6 baby or Persian cucumbers, washed, trimmed, and halved lengthwise, for serving

2 cups (182 grams) broccoli or cauliflower florets, for serving

DIRECTIONS

1 In a food processor, place the chickpeas (reserving 5 chickpeas for serving), the ice cube, 1 tablespoon of the olive oil, the lemon juice, the garlic, and the tahini sauce. Process for 2 to 3 minutes without stopping. Remove the lid and check the consistency. If it's too thick or it hasn't yet formed a paste, add water, 1 tablespoon (15 milliliters) at a time, until the mixture resembles a thick dip but is completely smooth. Season with salt and pepper, if needed.

2 Spoon the hummus onto a serving platter. Use the back of the spoon to create indentations in the hummus. Fill the holes with the remaining 3 tablespoons (45 milliliters) of olive oil. Place the remaining 5 chickpeas in the middle. Garnish with paprika and serve with the vegetable crudités.

PER SERVING: *Calories 295 (From Fat 109); Fat 12g (Saturated 2g); Cholesterol 0mg; Sodium 62mg; Carbohydrate 37g (Dietary Fiber 11g); Protein 12g.*

TIP: Traditional hummus should not have lumps. Peeling the chickpeas and adding an ice cube to the mix is an old Arab tradition that helps to maintain the smoothest texture possible.

NOTE: You'll need a good food processor with a sharp blade (or two) to create the right consistency. Most blenders are not powerful enough to achieve the right consistency.

VARY IT! The word *hummus* means chickpea in Arabic, so we don't recommend making the recipe with other beans. From a taste perspective, it still works with white beans or fava, but we would then call the recipe White Bean Puree or Fava Bean Puree. It's traditional to serve browned ground meat or shredded rotisserie chicken on top, too.

Hearty Main Courses

Making satisfying and tasty main courses that are known to manage cholesterol isn't difficult. By choosing to combine lots of fresh and green leafy vegetables with whole grains, lean proteins, beans and legumes, extra-virgin olive oil, herbs, and spices, you can create delicious dishes that are as good for your health as they are pleasing to your taste buds.

Luckily, heritage diets from all over the world offer a multitude of healthful choices with recipes that have stood the test of time. The recipes in this section feature fish, vegetables, lentils, and beans, with barley, brown rice, brown rice noodles, and heirloom pasta, along with vegetables that have an LDL cholesterol lowering effect. They're full of flavor, a joy to prepare, and fun to share with others.

TIP

To cut down on preparation time and make the process go smoother, read the recipe thoroughly a few times before preparing it. Make sure that you have all ingredients on hand in advance, and try the recipe out on yourself before preparing it for others. This way, you can make sure that it turns out the way you like it when serving it to others.

The recipes in this section were made to be enjoyed at more than one meal — you can make large batches and freeze them or store them in the refrigerator to be eaten at other times. They're flexible and easy to change. Be sure to look for a Vary It! paragraph at the bottom of the recipe to see suggestions.

Marinated Salmon and Brussels Sprouts over Citrus Cream Sauce

PREP TIME: ABOUT 15 MIN PLUS 30 MIN MARINATING	COOK TIME: 25 MIN	YIELD: 4 SERVINGS

INGREDIENTS

3 oranges (¼ cup [60 milliliters] freshly squeezed orange juice and zest, 1 orange sliced)

2 tablespoons (27 grams) extra-virgin olive oil

½ teaspoon (2 grams) unrefined sea salt

¼ teaspoon (1 gram) freshly ground black pepper

Four 4-ounce (113 grams) salmon fillets, skin on

2 cups (176 grams) Brussels sprouts, trimmed and cut into quarters

1 cup (240 grams) plain, full-fat Greek yogurt

DIRECTIONS

1 In a small bowl, whisk together the orange juice, olive oil, salt, and pepper until emulsified. Place the salmon fillets in a glass baking dish, and pour the dressing over the top. Cover with plastic and allow to marinate for 30 minutes in the refrigerator.

2 Preheat the oven to 425°F (218°C). Scatter the Brussels sprouts around the sides of the salmon. Bake until the fish flakes and the Brussels sprouts are tender, about 20 to 30 minutes.

3 While the fish is baking, combine the Greek yogurt and orange zest. To serve, place the yogurt mixture on the bottom of a serving platter, place the fish on top, and scatter the Brussels sprouts along the sides. Garnish each fish fillet and the dish with orange slices. Serve hot.

PER SERVING: *Calories 327 (From Fat 153); Fat 17g (Saturated 4g); Cholesterol 62mg; Sodium 317mg; Carbohydrate 14g (Dietary Fiber 2g); Protein 30g.*

TIP: Prepare the Brussels sprouts and make the yogurt sauce a day in advance for quicker prep.

NOTE: Leftovers taste great served over cooked barley, whole-wheat couscous or bulgur wheat.

VARY IT! You can use your favorite fish or chicken breast instead of salmon, if preferred. Replace the Brussels sprouts with broccoli, cauliflower, or fennel if you want.

Herb-Roasted "Plaki"-Style Fish with Vegetables and Brown Rice Pilaf

PREP TIME: ABOUT 15 MIN	COOK TIME: 50 MIN	YIELD: 6 SERVINGS

INGREDIENTS

¼ cup (54 grams) plus
1 teaspoon (5 grams) extra-virgin olive oil, divided

4 medium Yukon gold potatoes (about 2 pounds or 907 grams), cut into small wedges

3 green bell peppers, sliced into rings

2 zucchini, diced

3 medium tomatoes, diced

3 garlic cloves, peeled and sliced

1 bunch fresh parsley, washed, dried, and finely chopped, divided

1 bunch fresh baby dill, washed, dried, and finely chopped, divided

1 teaspoon (5 grams) unrefined sea salt, divided

½ teaspoon (1 gram) freshly ground black pepper

Six 4-ounce (115 grams) fish fillets (cod, red snapper, sea bass, halibut, or your favorite)

2 lemons, 1 sliced in half, the other cut into 6 slices

1 cup (185 grams) brown rice, rinsed

1 small onion, finely diced

2 cups (500 milliliters) Homemade Vegetable Stock (see Chapter 13)

DIRECTIONS

1 Preheat the oven to 425°F (218°C). Grease the bottom of an 11-x-17-inch baking pan with 1 teaspoon of the extra-virgin olive oil. Place the potatoes, peppers, tomatoes, zucchini, and garlic in the pan. Stir a handful of the chopped parsley and chopped dill into the vegetables, reserving the rest for the pilaf. Stir to combine. Season with ½ teaspoon (2 grams) of the salt and ¼ teaspoon (1 gram) of the pepper. Bake until the vegetables begin to soften, about 25 minutes.

2 Place the fish on top of the vegetables. Season with ¼ teaspoon (1 gram) of the salt and the remaining ¼ teaspoon (1 gram) of pepper. Drizzle the juice of the halved lemon over the top. Pour 3 tablespoons olive oil over the entire mixture. Stir to coat the vegetables under the fish. Bake until the fish flakes easily and the vegetables are cooked through, about 20 to 25 minutes.

3 Over medium heat, heat 1 tablespoon (14 grams) of the olive oil in a medium pot with a fitted lid. Add the onion and sauté until golden, 3 to 5 minutes. Add the brown rice and stir to coat. Stir in the remaining ¼ teaspoon (1 gram) of the salt. Add the vegetable stock and bring to a boil over high heat. Reduce the heat to low, cover, and cook until the pilaf is tender, about 40 to 50minutes. Remove from the heat and stir in the remaining parsley and dill.

4 Serve the fish and vegetables with brown rice while warm.

PER SERVING: *Calories 522 (From Fat 126); Fat 14g (Saturated 2g); Cholesterol 36mg; Sodium 559mg; Carbohydrate 68g (Dietary Fiber 7g); Protein 32g.*

TIP: The Greek term *plaki* means flat stone, and it refers to something baked in the oven. Chop the vegetables and roast them in advance, if desired, for quicker preparation.

NOTE: You can double this recipe to use the leftovers for other meals. You can make wraps, sandwiches, or even tacos using whole-wheat bread and tortillas with leftovers as well.

VARY IT! Use chicken breasts or tofu instead of fish.

🍅 Vegetable Stir-Fry with Edamame and Brown Rice Noodles

PREP TIME: ABOUT 15 MIN	COOK TIME: 10 MIN	YIELD: 4 SERVINGS

INGREDIENTS

2 tablespoons (27 grams) expeller-pressed sesame oil

1 bunch fresh asparagus, trimmed and cut into 3-inch (8-centimeter) pieces

2 cups (182 grams) broccoli florets

2 red peppers, thinly sliced

16 ounces (453 grams) frozen shelled edamame, thawed

3 cloves garlic, mined

1½ tablespoons (24 grams) low-sodium tamari

¼ cup (85 grams) raw honey

1 tablespoon (16 grams) almond butter

¼ cup (38 grams) raw sesame seeds

One 8-ounce (228 grams) package brown rice noodles

DIRECTIONS

1 In a large, wide skillet, heat the sesame oil over medium-high heat.

2 Add the asparagus, broccoli, peppers, and edamame and brown on all sides.

3 In a small bowl, combine the garlic, tamari, honey, almond butter, ½ cup (237 milliliters) water, and sesame seeds. Pour the mixture over the vegetable and edamame mixture and reduce the heat to medium-low, and allow them to simmer, stirring occasionally, until everything is slightly crunchy but tender inside, about 10 to 15 minutes.

4 Prepare the brown rice noodles according to package directions. Drain and toss them into the vegetable mixture. Turn with tongs to coat. Serve warm, immediately, or allow to cool and chill in the refrigerator to enjoy as a cold salad.

PER SERVING: *Calories 599 (From Fat 183); Fat 20g (Saturated 3g); Cholesterol 0mg; Sodium 414mg; Carbohydrate 89g (Dietary Fiber 12g); Protein 20g.*

TIP: We like to prepare large batches of this dish to enjoy as a cold salad for quick meals on the go.

NOTE: You can cook the vegetables a day in advance and toss them with the hot noodles before serving.

VARY IT! Swap out the edamame for 2 packages tempeh, fried eggs, or leftover cooked chicken breast or fish fillet, if desired.

🍅 Barley and Red Wine "Risotto" with Red Cabbage and Cannellini Beans

PREP TIME: ABOUT 10 MIN	COOK TIME: 40 MIN	YIELD: 6 SERVINGS

INGREDIENTS

¼ cup (54 grams) extra-virgin olive oil

1 shallot, finely minced

1 head red cabbage, trimmed, leaves roughly chopped

2 cups (400 grams) pearl barley

1 cup (235 grams) red wine

4½ cups (1 liter) Homemade Vegetable Stock (see Chapter 13)

¼ cup (20 grams) Parmigiano-Reggiano cheese

¼ teaspoon (1 gram) unrefined sea salt, if needed

1 cup (177 grams) Cannellini Beans (see Chapter 13)

¼ teaspoon (1 gram) freshly ground black pepper

1 small bunch fresh parsley, washed, dried, and finely chopped

DIRECTIONS

1 In a large pot, heat the extra-virgin olive oil over medium-high heat. Add the shallot, and cook until lightly golden and tender, approximately 3 to 5 minutes, stirring often. Add the cabbage, stir, and allow to cook until wilted, about 5 minutes.

2 Add the barley, and stir to coat well. Pour in the wine. Increase the heat to high, stir, and allow the alcohol to evaporate. Reduce the heat to medium, and add the stock, a ladleful at a time, until the barely is tender, about 30 minutes.

3 Stir in the cheese and taste. Add salt if needed. Stir in the beans and pepper.

4 To serve, place the barley on serving plates. Garnish with chopped parsley, and serve immediately.

PER SERVING: *Calories 428 (From Fat 99); Fat 11g (Saturated 2g); Cholesterol 2mg; Sodium 326mg; Carbohydrate 67g (Dietary Fiber 15g); Protein 12g.*

TIP: In Italy, it's fashionable to cook barley in the same manner, as carnaroli and arborio rice are used to make risotto. We love this version, which is easy on the digestion and great for lowering LDL cholesterol.

NOTE: If you already have cooked barley on hand, you could save time by sautéing the cabbage in a bit of extra-virgin olive oil and red wine and stirring it into the precooked barley with the beans and parsley.

VARY IT! Use cooked lentils instead of the beans in this dish if desired.

☝ Italian Pasta with Creamy Lentils and Pecorino Cheese

PREP TIME: ABOUT 10 MIN	COOK TIME: 15 MIN	YIELD: 6 SERVINGS

INGREDIENTS

¼ teaspoon (1 gram) unrefined sea salt

One 1-pound (454 grams) package whole-wheat or whole-grain pasta

¼ cup (54 grams) extra-virgin olive oil

1 large yellow onion, thinly sliced

1 recipe brown Lentils (see Chapter 13)

1 cup (246 grams) whole-milk ricotta cheese

¼ cup (25 grams) grated pecorino cheese, plus extra, for garnish, if desired.

1 bunch fresh parsley, finely chopped

¼ teaspoon (1 gram) freshly ground black pepper

DIRECTIONS

1 Bring a large pot of water to a boil over high heat. Add the salt and cook the pasta according to the package directions or until desired doneness. Reserve ½ cup (118 milliliters) of pasta water from cooking.

2 While the pasta is cooking, add the extra-virgin olive oil to a large wide skillet over medium-high heat. Add the onion, stir to coat, and reduce the heat to medium. Sauté the onion until it becomes translucent and slightly golden in color, about 10 minutes.

3 Place the lentils in a food processor or blender and puree until smooth. Add the pureed lentils, ricotta, pecorino, and parsley to a heat-proof bowl. Stir in the hot pasta water. Drain the pasta and place back in the pot. Stir in the lentil mixture. Add the pepper, top with additional pecorino cheese, if desired, and serve immediately.

PER SERVING: *Calories 563 (From Fat 153); Fat 17g (Saturated 6g); Cholesterol 25mg; Sodium 267mg; Carbohydrate 82g (Dietary Fiber 10g); Protein 26g.*

TIP: Keep caramelized or sautéed onions on hand in the refrigerator to add flavor and nutrition to meals. When possible, make the base recipes in Chapter 13 and keep them in the refrigerator for up to a week to use when needed.

NOTE: You can leave the lentils whole and omit the pureeing, if desired.

VARY IT! Make the same dish with brown rice and/or swap the lentils for your favorite legumes.

Satisfying Salads

Salads are known for being healthful, but often they're less appreciated for their flavors and ability to fill you up. When they're trying to eat well, many people include the same simple green or mixed salads in their meals. There's nothing wrong with that approach, but if you consistently rely on the same recipe, you'll easily get bored with its taste and likely crave more unhealthful foods instead. To get the most taste and nutrition out of salad recipes, be sure to create them with the same amount of inspiration as you would any other recipe.

The salads in this section rely on a wide range of fruits and vegetables to provide a variety of nutrients and delicious tastes. You can enjoy the salads as is, along with the appetizers or main dishes in this chapter, or enhance them — see the Tip paragraphs for ideas to transform these salads into one-dish meals.

A key element to maximizing the nutrition quotient of a salad is dressing it properly. These recipes use good-quality extra-virgin olive oil and antioxidant-rich citrus juice and herbs, along with probiotic-packed vinegars in place of fat-, sugar-, and sodium-ladened bottled dressings in order to turn them into tasty culinary medicine.

Because salads wilt when stored with dressing already mixed in, we recommend making large batches of each to have on hand for a few days and storing them with dressings apart until serving. This will enable you to save time and enjoy the fiber-rich foods that are so important for managing cholesterol whenever hunger strikes.

Red Cabbage, Citrus, and Carrot Slaw with Cilantro Vinaigrette

PREP TIME: ABOUT 15 MIN	COOK TIME: NONE	YIELD: 8 SERVINGS

INGREDIENTS

1 head red cabbage, trimmed and shredded

4 mandarin oranges, peeled and sliced into segments

4 carrots, peeled, trimmed, and shredded

¼ cup (54 grams) extra-virgin olive oil

Juice of 1 lemon

Juice of 1 orange

1 bunch fresh cilantro, washed and dried

1 teaspoon (7 grams) raw honey

¼ teaspoon (1 gram) unrefined sea salt

¼ teaspoon (1 gram) freshly ground black pepper

DIRECTIONS

1 In a large bowl, place the cabbage, oranges, and carrots.

2 In a blender, combine the extra-virgin olive oil, lemon juice, orange juice, cilantro, honey, salt, and pepper and whip on high to emulsify. If you prefer, you can whisk the ingredients in a bowl until a homogeneous dressing is formed.

3 Pour the dressing over the salad, toss to coat, and serve immediately.

PER SERVING: *Calories 123 (From Fat 64); Fat 7g (Saturated 1g); Cholesterol 0mg; Sodium 100mg; Carbohydrate 16g (Dietary Fiber 3g); Protein 2g.*

TIP: Add leftover fish, smoked salmon, or cannellini beans to turn this salad into a light meal.

VARY IT! Use Italian parsley instead of cilantro, if you prefer.

Artichoke, Pea, and Cherry Tomato Salad with Lemon and Basil Dressing

PREP TIME: ABOUT 15 MIN	COOK TIME: 20 MIN	YIELD: 4 SERVINGS

INGREDIENTS

8 cooked Baby Artichokes (see Chapter 13) or frozen artichokes, thawed* (See Tip)

2 cups (320 grams) sugar snap peas, trimmed (see Tip)

1 cup (149 grams) cherry tomatoes, halved

1 tablespoon (15 grams) Dijon mustard

Juice and zest of 2 lemons

¼ teaspoon (1 gram) unrefined sea salt

⅛ teaspoon (1 gram) freshly ground black pepper

2 tablespoons (27 gram) extra-virgin olive oil

¼ cup (6 grams) finely chopped fresh basil

DIRECTIONS

1 In a large bowl, combine the artichokes, snap peas, and cherry tomatoes.

2 In a medium bowl, whisk together the mustard, lemon juice and zest, salt, and pepper. Once combined, whisk in the olive oil until an emulsified dressing is formed. Stir in the basil.

3 Pour the dressing over the salad, toss to, and serve immediately.

PER SERVING: *Calories 193 (From Fat 68); Fat 8g (Saturated 1g); Cholesterol 0mg; Sodium 503mg; Carbohydrate 28g (Dietary Fiber 12g); Protein 9g.*

TIP: When in season, fresh artichokes are delicious. If you can't find them fresh, you can usually find frozen versions in supermarkets and online.

TIP: To trim snap peas, snip the stem to remove it. Then peel away the string that runs along the pod by pulling it. Open the pod and remove the peas.

NOTE: The artichoke, pea, and cherry tomato combination also makes a great condiment for pasta. Just toss hot, whole-wheat or whole-grain pasta with the vegetables, add basil and extra-virgin olive oil.

VARY IT! To turn this salad into a full meal, add quartered hard-boiled eggs or edamame to the recipe.

🍅 Spinach, Lentil, and Pomegranate Salad

PREP TIME: ABOUT 15 MIN	COOK TIME: NONE	YIELD: 4 SERVINGS

INGREDIENTS

1 cup (198 grams) Brown Lentils (see Chapter 13)

4 cups (120 grams) baby spinach

Arils and juice of 2 ripe pomegranates (about 1 cup [174 grams] arils and ½ cup [125 grams] juice) (see Tip)

1 teaspoon (6 grams) pomegranate molasses

2 tablespoons (27 grams) extra-virgin olive oil

¼ teaspoon (1 gram) unrefined sea salt

¼ teaspoon (1 gram) freshly ground black pepper

DIRECTIONS

1 In a large bowl, combine the lentils, spinach, and pomegranate arils.

2 In a medium bowl, combine the pomegranate juice, pomegranate molasses, extra-virgin olive oil, salt, and pepper. Whisk well until emulsified and pour over the salad. Toss to coat.

PER SERVING: *Calories 182 (From Fat 69); Fat 8g (Saturated 1g); Cholesterol 0mg; Sodium 146mg; Carbohydrate 25g (Dietary Fiber 6g); Protein 6g.*

TIP: Only make this salad when pomegranates are in season. When purchasing pomegranates, it's important to note that the ones that look less attractive on the outside are usually the sweetest and contain the most juice. To use, cut the pomegranate in half. Squeeze juice out through a strainer into a bowl. Place the pomegranate shell and strained arils into a bowl of water and gently pull the sections apart under the water. Loosen and separate the arils with your fingers. The white pith will float to the surface. Skim it off the top and discard it. Drain the arils and use them.

NOTE: You can find pomegranate molasses at Middle Eastern markets and specialty stores. If you can't find it, you can order it online or make your own by cooking down ¼ cup (62 grams) pomegranate juice until it forms a thick syrup.

VARY IT! To make this salad a meal, add pieces of cooked rotisserie chicken, leg of lamb, or creamy goat cheese and walnuts.

Moroccan Carrot Salad

PREP TIME: ABOUT 15 MIN	COOK TIME: NONE	YIELD: 4 SERVINGS

INGREDIENTS

3 cups (330 grams) shredded carrots

2 navel oranges, peeled and cut into segments

1 bunch fresh parsley, washed, dried, and finely chopped

8 plump Medjool dates, pitted and sliced into quarters (see Tip)

Juice of 1 orange

Juice of 1 lemon

1 teaspoon (5 milliliters) orange blossom water

¼ teaspoon (1 gram) freshly ground black pepper

DIRECTIONS

1 In a large bowl, combine the carrots, oranges, parsley, and dates.

2 In a medium bowl, whisk together the orange juice, lemon juice, and orange blossom water. Add the black pepper, and whisk to form an emulsified dressing.

3 Pour the dressing over the salad, toss to coat, and spoon onto a serving platter in a pyramid shape to serve.

PER SERVING: *Calories 210 (From Fat 4); Fat 0g (Saturated 0g); Cholesterol 0mg; Sodium 58mg; Carbohydrate 55g (Dietary Fiber 7g); Protein 2g.*

TIP: Keep shredded carrots in the fridge to make preparing this salad a cinch. If your dates are very dry, soak them in water for 15 to 20 minutes to plump them.

NOTE: Orange blossom water adds a lovely fragrance and depth of flavor to Moroccan recipes. You can find it in Middle Eastern markets or online. Omit it if you don't have it on hand.

VARY IT! Add grilled chicken to this salad to turn it into a one-dish meal.

⊙ Avocado, Citrus, and Spinach Salad with Walnuts and White Balsamic Vinaigrette

PREP TIME: ABOUT 15 MIN	COOK TIME: 10 MIN	YIELD: 6 SERVINGS

INGREDIENTS

8 ounces (227 grams) romaine, cut into bite-size pieces

2 large oranges, trimmed and cut into segments

1 large ripe tomato, cut into 13 equal pieces

2 ripe avocados, pitted, peeled, and diced

½ cup (60 grams) walnut pieces, toasted and cooled (see Tip)

3 tablespoons (41 grams) extra-virgin olive oil

2 tablespoons (32 grams) white balsamic vinegar

¼ teaspoon (1 gram) unrefined sea salt

¼ teaspoon (1 gram) freshly ground black pepper

DIRECTIONS

1 In a large bowl, place the romaine, oranges, tomato, avocado and walnuts. Toss to combine.

2 In a medium bowl, combine the extra-virgin olive oil, vinegar, salt, and pepper. Whisk well until emulsified. Toss with the salad and serve.

PER SERVING: *Calories 269 (From Fat 210); Fat 23g (Saturated 3g); Cholesterol 0mg; Sodium 89mg; Carbohydrate 16g (Dietary Fiber 7g); Protein 4g.*

TIP: Toasting nuts brings out their flavor. To toast walnuts, place them on a baking sheet and bake at 375°F (191°C) for 5 to 10 minutes or until they begin to release their aroma. Allow to cool before using.

VARY IT! Add your favorite cooked fish or quinoa to this recipe to turn the salad into a complete meal. Use baby kale, dandelion greens, spinach, or mixed field greens instead of the romaine lettuce if you prefer.

Dazzling Desserts

Desserts are probably the last thing that come to your mind when thinking about managing cholesterol. Not all desserts are created equal, and most commonly prepared desserts should be enjoyed on very rare occasions and with extreme caution. That's because many of them are full of butter or margarine, sugar, other fats, and ingredients known for increasing LDL cholesterol.

The desserts in this section, however, are made with fresh fruit, such as apples, grapes, strawberries, blueberries, and citrus, all of which contain powerful antioxidants that have a positive effect on cholesterol. They also include whole grains, which are full of fiber; use extra-virgin olive oil as the main fat source; and incorporate polyphenol-rich dark chocolate and red wine. Each of these desserts is as delicious as it is good for you.

Be sure to read the tip following each recipe to learn how to make the recipe in advance to cut down on preparation time. By having desserts like this on hand or already prepared in the freezer, you can prevent yourself from derailing your eating plan with more unhealthful sweet treats.

🍅 Individual Spiced Apple Pies with Almond and Oatmeal Crust

PREP TIME: ABOUT 20 MIN	COOK TIME: 30 MIN PLUS 1 HR CHILLING	YIELD: 5 SERVINGS

INGREDIENTS

2 cups (324 grams) oat flour

½ cup (41 grams) whole oats

⅓ cup (71 grams) plus 1 teaspoon (5 grams) extra-virgin olive oil, divided

⅓ cup (66 grams) plus 2 tablespoons (25 grams) sugar, divided

4 apples, cored, and cut into 8 slices each

1 lemon, juiced and zested

1 cinnamon stick

½ teaspoon (1 gram) ground cloves

1 teaspoon (4 grams) vanilla extract

3 tablespoons (21 grams) cornstarch, diluted in ¼ cup (59 milliliters) water

1 egg white, lightly beaten

DIRECTIONS

1 In a food processor fitted with a metal blade, combine the flour, oats, and 1/3 cup (71 grams) of the extra-virgin olive oil until crumbly in texture. Add the egg, 2 tablespoons (25 grams) of the sugar, and 4 tablespoons (59 milliliters) water. Mix the dough until it's completely softened and begins to form a ball. Work into a ball, cover, and refrigerate 1 hour.

2 Prepare the filling: In a medium saucepan, combine the apple slices, lemon juice, cinnamon stick, cloves, and vanilla. Add the remaining ⅓ cup (71 grams) sugar and the cornstarch mixture and mix to coat. Bring to a boil over medium heat, reduce the heat to low stirring slowly and continue to cook until the mixture resembles a pie filling, about 3 to 5 minutes.

3 When the dough has been chilled, preheat the oven to 400°F (204°C). Grease five 4-inch (10-centimeter) tart pans with the remaining 1 teaspoon of olive oil. Roll the dough out onto a 12-inch (31-centimeter) circle. Use the mini tart pans as cookie cutters to cut out 5 circles in the dough (scraping up and rerolling extra dough if necessary). Press the dough down into the tart shells and prick them with a fork. Line with parchment paper. Fill with pie weights, rice, or dried beans to help the crusts maintain their shape while baking. Bake until slightly golden, about 20 minutes.

4 Remove from the oven. Remove the parchment paper and weights. Brush the crust with egg white and return to the oven for 10 minutes. Let cool slightly and carefully remove the crusts from the pan. Fill each one with the apple filling and garnish with lemon zest to serve.

PER SERVING: *Calories 597 (From Fat 197); Fat 22g (Saturated 3g); Cholesterol 0mg; Sodium 27mg; Carbohydrate 91g (Dietary Fiber 9g); Protein 12g.*

TIP: You can make the pie shells up to a month in advance and store them in an airtight container in the freezer. Bring to room temperature before filling.

NOTE: You can use the same recipe to make a 10-inch (25-centimeter) open-faced pie.

VARY IT! Use mixed berries instead of apples, if desired.

🍅 Italian Grape Harvest Cake with Cinnamon–Red Wine Reduction

PREP TIME: ABOUT 10 MIN	COOK TIME: 45 MIN	YIELD: 9 SERVINGS

INGREDIENTS

½ cup (108 grams) plus 2 teaspoons (9 grams) extra-virgin olive oil, divided

½ cup (53 grams) sliced almonds

2 eggs, separated

⅔ cup (164 grams) freshly squeezed orange juice

2 teaspoons (4 grams) grated orange zest

1 cup (200 grams) sugar

2 teaspoons (8 grams) vanilla extract

2⅓ cups (261 grams) almond flour

1 teaspoon (2 grams) baking powder

½ teaspoon (1 gram) unrefined sea salt

1 cup (151 grams) red grapes

2 cups (454 grams) red wine

1 cinnamon stick

DIRECTIONS

1 Preheat the oven to 350°F (177°C). Grease (with 1 teaspoon [0.33 gram] of the extra-virgin olive oil) and flour a 9-inch (23-centimeter) springform pan. Line with parchment paper. Brush the parchment paper with 1 teaspoon (0.33 gram) of the olive oil and sprinkle with sliced almonds.

2 In the bowl of a standing mixer or in a large metal bowl using a hand mixer, beat the egg whites until stiff peaks form. Set aside.

3 In a separate bowl, combine the orange juice, orange zest, the remaining ½ cup (108 grams) olive oil, egg yolks, sugar, and vanilla.

4 In a large bowl, sift together the flour, baking powder, and salt in the orange juice mixture, and fold in the grapes and the egg whites.

5 Pour the batter into the prepared pan, and smooth out the top with a spatula. Bake until a toothpick inserted into the middle comes out clean and the cake begins to pull away from the sides of the pan, about 40 to 45 minutes.

6 While the cake is baking, place the wine and cinnamon stick in a medium saucepan. Bring to boil over high heat. Reduce the heat to low and simmer until the mixture is condensed and syrupy in consistency, about 20 to 30 minutes. Set aside to cool.

7 Cool the cake completely. Invert the cake onto a platter, and release the sides of the pan. Remove the parchment paper, and serve with wine reduction drizzled on top.

PER SERVING: *Calories 484 (From Fat 284); Fat 32g (Saturated 3g); Cholesterol 47mg; Sodium 98mg; Carbohydrate 36g (Dietary Fiber 5g); Protein 9g.*

TIP: If you'd like to pair this dessert with wine, look for *a passito,* Moscato, or similar.

NOTE: The extra-virgin olive oil is a beautiful compliment to the flavor and consistency of cakes.

VARY IT! You can use oat flour instead of almond flour, if you prefer, or a combination of them.

Decadent Dark Chocolate Mousse with Strawberries

PREP TIME: ABOUT 15 MIN	COOK TIME: 6 MIN PLUS OVERNIGHT CHILLING	YIELD: 8 SERVINGS

INGREDIENTS

8 ounces (227 grams) dark chocolate (at least 70% cacao)

3 large eggs (see Tip)

1 tablespoon (13 grams) vanilla extract

1 cup (238 grams) whipping cream, whipped until stiff

2 cups (288 grams) hulled strawberries, sliced

DIRECTIONS

1 Preheat the oven to 300°F (149°C).

2 Put the chocolate in a small ovenproof bowl or glass pan and place in the oven for a few minutes until the chocolate has melted, approximately 4 to 6 minutes. Remove from the oven and allow to cool until room temperature.

3 Beat the eggs until foamy. Whisk the eggs slowly into the cooled chocolate until incorporated. Stir in the vanilla, and fold in the whipped cream. Allow to chill overnight.

4 Divide the strawberries into 4 dessert bowls or cups. Using an ice cream scoop, spoon equal portions of the mousse onto each pile of strawberries. Serve immediately.

PER SERVING: *Calories 315 (From Fat 226); Fat 25g (Saturated 14g); Cholesterol 121mg; Sodium 44mg; Carbohydrate 17g (Dietary Fiber 4g); Protein 5g.*

TIP: The eggs in this recipe are not fully cooked. Use pasteurized eggs if you prefer, or do not consume if you have compromised health, are pregnant, or were instructed not to eat raw eggs by your healthcare professional.

NOTE: This mousse also makes a delicious cake filling.

🍅 Fresh Summer Berry Clafoutis

| PREP TIME: ABOUT 10 MIN | COOK TIME: 20 MIN | YIELD: 4 SERVINGS |

INGREDIENTS

½ teaspoon (2 grams) extra-virgin olive oil

5 tablespoons (63 grams) sugar, divided

2 extra-large eggs

½ cup (56 grams) almond flour

1 cup (227 grams) plain, full-fat Greek yogurt

1 tablespoon (13 grams) vanilla extract

1 teaspoon (2 grams) orange zest

1 teaspoon (4 grams) almond extract

Pinch unrefined sea salt

1 cup (148 grams) mixed berries

DIRECTIONS

1 Preheat the oven to 375°F (191°C). Grease an 8-inch (20-centimeter) baking dish with extra-virgin olive oil. Sprinkle 2 tablespoons (25 grams) sugar over the bottom.

2 Beat the eggs and the remaining 3 tablespoons (38 grams) sugar in the bowl of an electric mixer fitted with the paddle attachment on medium-high speed until foamy. Add in the flour, yogurt, vanilla, orange zest, almond extract, and salt.

3 Add the berries to the bottom of the baking dish. Turn to coat in the sugar and pour the batter over the top. Bake until the top is golden and the custard is set, about 15 to 20 minutes. Serve warm.

PER SERVING: *Calories 271 (From Fat 118); Fat 13g (Saturated 3g); Cholesterol 118mg; Sodium 89mg; Carbohydrate 28g (Dietary Fiber 3g); Protein 12g.*

TIP: Clafoutis is an old French staple and an easy dessert to whip up when you have unexpected guests.

NOTE: In this recipe, the traditional heavy cream is replaced with the healthier Greek yogurt.

VARY IT! You can substitute peaches or plums for the berries when in season. Swap almond flour for oat flour or unbleached all-purpose flour, if you want.

Orange and Olive Oil Walnut Cake

PREP TIME: ABOUT 15 MIN | **COOK TIME: 30 MIN** | **YIELD: 8 SERVINGS**

INGREDIENTS

¼ cup (54 grams) plus 1 teaspoon (5 grams) extra-virgin olive oil, divided

⅔ cup (107 grams) oat flour

2 teaspoons (9 grams) baking powder

Grated zest and juice of 2 oranges, separated

¼ teaspoon (1 gram) unrefined sea salt

4 large eggs, separated, divided

½ cup (100 grams) sugar

1 teaspoon (4 grams) vanilla extract

1 cup (100 grams) walnuts, toasted and chopped, divided

1 tablespoon (8 grams) powdered sugar, for garnish

DIRECTIONS

1 Preheat the oven to 350°F (177°C). Using 1 teaspoon (5 grams) of the olive oil, grease a 9-inch (23-centimeter) springform pan; dust it with flour.

2 In a small bowl, mix the flour, baking powder, orange zest, and salt.

3 In another bowl, beat the egg yolks and sugar together until thick and pale yellow, about 3 minutes. Slowly add in the remaining ¼ cup (54 grams) of olive oil, the orange juice, and the vanilla. Stir in the flour mixture and ½ cup (50g) of the walnuts.

4 Using clean beaters, in a separate metal bowl, beat the egg whites until stiff peaks form. Stir the egg whites into the batter until no white is visible. Transfer the batter to the prepared pan. Top with the remaining ½ cup (50 grams) of walnuts. Place the pan in the center of the oven and bake until a toothpick inserted into the center comes out clean, about 25 to 30 minutes.

5 Cool the cake in the pan on a rack. Place the cake on a platter and garnish with powdered sugar.

PER SERVING: *Calories 300 (From Fat 173); Fat 19g (Saturated 3g); Cholesterol 106mg; Sodium 219mg; Carbohydrate 27g (Dietary Fiber 2g); Protein 7g.*

TIP: Toasting walnuts brings out their flavor. To toast, place walnuts on a baking sheet in a 350°F (177°C) oven. Toast until they release their aroma, about 5 to 10 minutes. Allow to cool completely and chop finely.

TIP: You can make this cake in advance and store it for up to a month in the freezer.

VARY IT! Add chopped dates, raisins, or dried apricots to this cake, if you want.

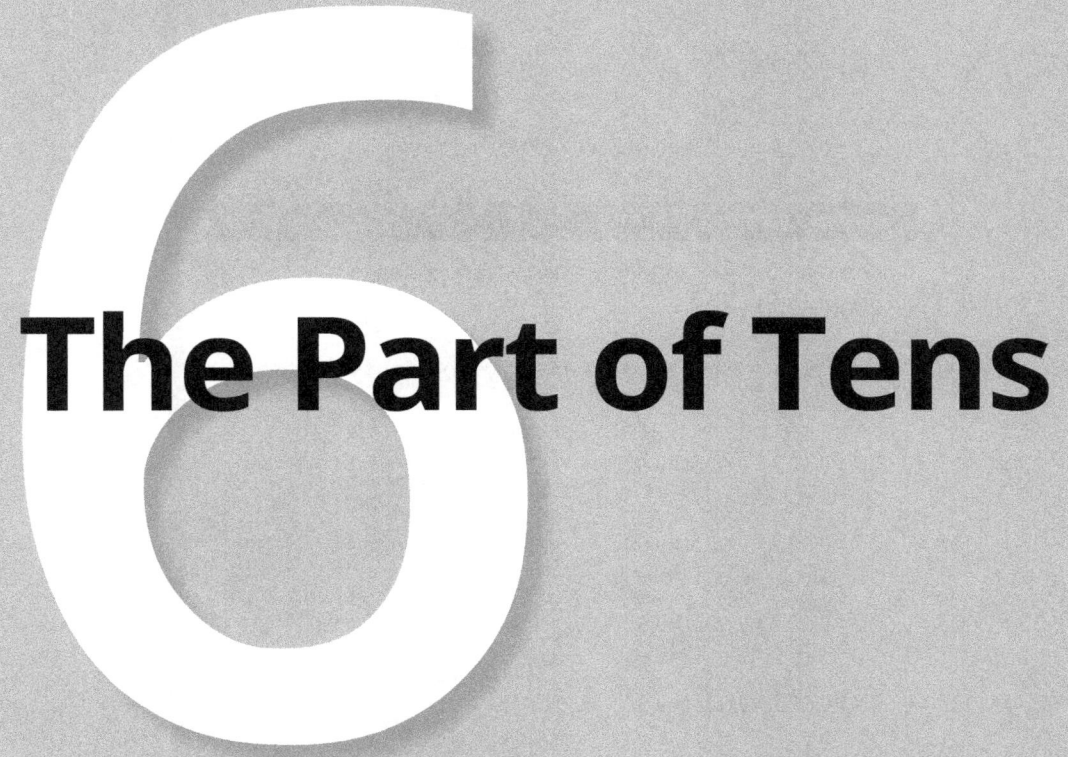

The Part of Tens

IN THIS PART . . .

Discover ten easy and effective ways to manage cholesterol.

Incorporate ten cholesterol-friendly foods into your diet.

Learn ten misconceptions about cholesterol.

IN THIS CHAPTER

» Starting your cholesterol
management journey

» Appreciating some quick, easy wins

» Finding inspiring, positive, and simple
new approaches to cholesterol
management

Chapter **16**

Ten Easy Wins to Manage Cholesterol

The processes driving high cholesterol, its oxidation, and the laying down of plaque resulting in inflammation, arteriosclerosis, and cardiovascular disease (CVD) are complex. Accurately assessing an individual person's risk of developing CVD is also not straightforward, especially when influential lifestyle factors are difficult to measure.

There are, however several simple ways in which you can reduce your cholesterol and also decrease the likelihood of any given level of cholesterol driving plaque formation and progress to CVD.

In this chapter, you find some simple yet highly effective ways to rapidly and positively impact your cholesterol management.

Increasing Your Fiber Intake

Increasing your fiber intake is a powerful strategy to help manage cholesterol levels. Dietary fiber, especially soluble fiber, binds to cholesterol in the digestive system and supports its removal from the body before it enters the bloodstream.

TIP

To increase fiber intake, start by adding more whole, plant-based foods to your daily diet. Fruits such as apples, berries, and pears are excellent sources of soluble fiber, as are vegetables like Brussels sprouts and carrots. Legumes, including beans, chickpeas, and lentils, are fiber powerhouses that you can easily add to soups or salads or eat as a side dish. Whole grains, like barley, brown rice, and oats, also contribute significant amounts of fiber. Making small, gradual changes can help prevent digestive discomfort as your body adjusts. For example, swap white bread for whole-grain varieties, choose oatmeal instead of sugary cereals, and snack on nuts or fresh fruit rather than processed foods.

REMEMBER

Aim for a daily fiber intake of at least 25 to 30 grams, which you can achieve by incorporating these whole foods throughout the day. Drinking plenty of water also helps fiber move smoothly through your digestive system, enhancing its cholesterol-lowering benefits.

Choosing Healthy Fats

Choosing healthy fats is another essential step in managing cholesterol levels. Fats are an important part of the diet, but not all fats are created equal. Unsaturated fats, found in foods like avocados, nuts, and olive oil, can help lower low-density lipoprotein (LDL) cholesterol, often called "bad" cholesterol, while raising high-density lipoprotein (HDL) cholesterol, known as "good" cholesterol.

TIP

Incorporating these fats can be as simple as using extra-virgin olive oil instead of butter when cooking or dressing salads. Fatty fish, such as mackerel, salmon, and sardines, are rich in omega-3 fatty acids, which have been shown to lower triglycerides and improve heart health. Try to include fish in your meals at least twice a week for maximum benefit.

WARNING

Limit saturated fats, especially those that are found in processed and red meats and fried foods (other than those prepared in extra-virgin olive oil), because they can raise LDL cholesterol levels. Avoid trans fats altogether — they're commonly found in processed and packaged foods or in fried food restaurants using poor quality oils exposed to prolonged heating. They can significantly raise LDL cholesterol while lowering HDL cholesterol.

REMEMBER

By choosing heart-healthy fats and being mindful of your fat sources, you can make a substantial difference in your cholesterol levels.

Reading Food Labels

Reading food labels is a practical and empowering tool for controlling cholesterol. Nutrition labels provide crucial information about the fat content, fiber levels, and other key nutrients in packaged foods. When checking labels, pay close attention to the amount of saturated and trans fats, sometimes called "partially hydrogenated fats" — minimize your intake of saturated fat, and avoid trans fats completely.

Look for products that contain heart-healthy ingredients like whole grains and unsaturated fats while steering clear of added sugars and refined carbohydrates, which can contribute to weight gain and negatively affect cholesterol. Additives and preservatives in ultra-processed foods may have a detrimental effect on cholesterol levels, adversely affect your gut microbiome or increase oxidative stress. Look for simple, recognizable, natural ingredients — and if you like, turn to apps such as Yuka, which analyze the nutritional content of ingredients when you scan the product bar code.

REMEMBER

Taking a few extra minutes to review labels when grocery shopping can help you make smarter, heart-healthy choices and stay on track with your cholesterol management goals.

Focusing on a Sustainable Mediterranean Diet

Enjoying a Mediterranean diet will probably improve your cholesterol.

REMEMBER

Not everything that counts can be counted, and it's also likely that a Mediterranean diet will have an even greater beneficial effect on your levels of LDL cholesterol oxidation, oxidative stress in general, markers of inflammation, and other factors that contribute significantly to the development of arteriosclerosis and your risk of CVD. These factors are less easy to quantify in a simple blood test and are not directly measured or included in CVD risk score tools, so they may not be the focus of conversation when you discuss your cholesterol numbers with your doctor. Nevertheless, they're extremely important when it comes to protecting your health and increasing the likelihood of "adding years to life and life to years."

Plant-rich diets low in saturated fat have been shown to not only reduce cholesterol levels but also reverse the effects of arteriosclerosis. The Mediterranean diet is an excellent choice when it comes to managing cholesterol. The evidence for its positive effects is well established, it's an enjoyable and sustainable way to enjoy nutritious foods, and its protective effects against other conditions like many types of cancer, Alzheimer's disease, and numerous other chronic diseases is definitely an added advantage.

The Mediterranean diet is high in healthy fats, unrefined whole-grain carbohydrates, fiber-rich plant proteins with anti-inflammatory and antioxidant polyphenols (especially in the colored and flavorful vegetables, fruits, nuts, herbs, spices and extra-virgin olive oil). A diet with the highest intake of polyphenols has been shown to be associated with a 46 percent reduced risk of CVD.

REMEMBER

Nutrition experts say that the Mediterranean diet is the healthiest in the world, and with the detailed advice we offer in Chapter 6, making the switch has never been easier.

Embracing Extra-Virgin Olive Oil

Extra-virgin olive oil is a key ingredient in the Mediterranean diet as the most ubiquitous cooking oil and dressing for meals — it's so important that we wrote an entire book on the subject; *Olive Oil For Dummies* (John Wiley & Sons), which can certainly help you to appreciate and enjoy more of this extraordinarily healthful food.

REMEMBER

Research has shown that regular consumption of 2 tablespoons of extra-virgin olive oil per day as part of a Mediterranean diet has been shown to be associated with a reduction in heart disease, stroke, and mortality by more than 30 percent.

Olive oil is a healthy fat. It's high in the monounsaturated fat oleic acid, which has a beneficial effect on cholesterol levels. But the power of extra-virgin olive oil probably comes more from its ability to reduce the damaging oxidation of LDL cholesterol, crucial in the formation of the plaques of arteriosclerosis. These effects come from some unique and very special polyphenols found in some extra-virgin olive oils.

TIP

Not all olive oils are the same, and only a small proportion of those on supermarket shelves will meet the threshold of polyphenol levels that have a measurable effect in reducing oxidation of LDL cholesterol. The oil must be designated extra-virgin quality and, to preserve the precious polyphenols, it must have been produced with great care; harvested early; protected from light, heat, and air in storage; consumed fresh; and have the pleasant peppery and slightly bitter flavors that are signs of the presence of the most important polyphenols.

Planning Your Meals

Planning your meals is a simple yet effective strategy for managing cholesterol levels. When you plan ahead, you have greater control over the ingredients you use and the balance of nutrients in your diet. Start by incorporating heart-healthy foods such as fruits, vegetables, whole grains, and lean proteins according to the Mediterranean diet (or another heritage diet) into your weekly menu.

For instance, you may prepare a batch of vegetable soup or roasted vegetables at the start of the week to have on hand for easy, nutritious meals. Prioritize sources of healthy fats like extra-virgin olive oil, nuts, and fatty fish, while reducing processed foods that often contain high levels of saturated and trans fats, as well as other potentially unhelpful ingredients. Meal planning also allows you to control portion sizes, which can prevent overeating and help maintain a healthy weight.

When dining out, look for options that align with your heart-healthy choices, such as grilled instead of fried foods (unless you know they're freshly prepared in extra-virgin olive oil) and salads with olive oil–based dressings. By making meal planning a regular habit, you can avoid last-minute, less-healthy choices and keep your cholesterol in check.

For more information see Chapters 13 and 14, as well as our book *Diabetes Meal Planning & Nutrition For Dummies* (John Wiley & Sons), which focuses on diabetes but is very much aligned with meal planning for successful cholesterol management.

Enjoying More Exercise

Enjoying more exercise is another powerful way to improve cholesterol levels and overall heart health. Physical activity helps increase HDL cholesterol, the "good" cholesterol that helps remove harmful cholesterol from the bloodstream. You don't need to become a marathon runner to see benefits — small, consistent changes can have a significant impact.

TIP

Aim to incorporate at least 150 minutes of moderate exercise per week. Moderate exercise can be as simple as brisk walking, cycling, or dancing. Find activities you enjoy to make exercise feel less like a chore and more like a rewarding part of your day. If you're short on time, break exercise into shorter sessions — ten minutes of walking after meals can add up over time. Incorporating more movement into your daily routine, such as taking the stairs instead of the elevator or stretching during breaks, also contributes to better heart health. Regular exercise not only helps with cholesterol but also supports weight management, blood pressure control, and mental well-being, making it a crucial part of a heart-healthy lifestyle.

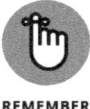

REMEMBER

Not everything that matters can be measured. Just as there are profound benefits beyond just the cholesterol number or risk calculator result by adopting a Mediterranean diet, regular exercise results in decreased oxidative stress and promotes an anti-inflammatory physiological state, which reduces the harmful potential of any given level of LDL cholesterol and enhances plaque stability.

Sleeping Well

Sleep is often overlooked, but it plays a critical role in maintaining healthy cholesterol levels. Poor sleep can disrupt your body's ability to regulate cholesterol and may increase the risk of heart disease over time. Aim for seven to nine hours of quality sleep each night to support overall health.

Establishing a consistent bedtime routine can improve sleep quality. This may include winding down with a book, practicing relaxation techniques, or limiting screen time before bed. Creating a restful sleep environment by keeping your bedroom cool, quiet, and dark can also promote better rest. Avoiding caffeine and heavy meals late in the evening can further enhance sleep. (Turn to Chapter 9 for more information.)

If you struggle with persistent sleep difficulties, consider discussing your concerns with a healthcare professional. Untreated sleep problems, such as sleep apnea, can contribute to cardiovascular risks. Prioritizing regular, restorative sleep not only supports cholesterol management but also improves mood, cognitive function, and overall vitality.

Taking Care of Yourself

Taking care of yourself may seem obvious, but few of us actually spend much time considering how best to deal with the stresses in our busy lives, nurturing relationships, and fostering emotional well-being, all of which can impact cholesterol levels. Chronic stress may trigger unhealthy coping mechanisms, such as overeating or choosing high-fat, sugary foods, which can elevate cholesterol. Stress itself can affect hormones, which more directly result in changes in circulating cholesterol.

Engaging in activities that promote relaxation, such as yoga, meditation, or spending time in nature, can help reduce stress levels and support heart health. Maintaining social connections is also important; whether through family gatherings, community activities, or simply keeping in touch with loved ones, these relationships can provide emotional support and reduce feelings of isolation.

REMEMBER

Prioritizing self-care means recognizing your mental and emotional needs alongside physical health. By cultivating a balanced lifestyle that includes regular rest, joyful activities, and supportive relationships, you can create an environment where both your mind and body thrive, contributing to healthier cholesterol levels.

Checking Out Other Risks for Cardiovascular Disease

Checking out other CVD risks is an essential step in managing your vascular health comprehensively and reducing the physical and chemical processes that result in cholesterol-forming plaques progressing to arteriosclerosis.

REMEMBER

Cholesterol itself is just one factor. Other risks, such as high blood pressure, diabetes, smoking, and a sedentary lifestyle, also play a significant role in damaging blood vessel walls or increasing oxidative stress, making the inner lining of blood vessels more likely to be breached by circulating cholesterol. Regular health checkups allow you to monitor these key indicators and catch potential issues early. Blood pressure measurements, blood sugar tests, and body mass index (BMI) assessments are simple but informative tests that can help you understand your overall risk profile.

If you have a family history of heart disease, sharing this information with your healthcare provider is important for assessing your personal risk. Lifestyle changes, such as eating a heart-healthy diet, exercising regularly, and avoiding tobacco products address multiple risk factors simultaneously. Being proactive about understanding and managing all aspects of cardiovascular health gives you the best chance of maintaining a healthy heart and reducing the long-term risks associated with elevated cholesterol.

Chapter **17**

Ten Cholesterol-Friendly Foods to Incorporate into Your Diet

C hoosing delicious foods to support how you manage your cholesterol is key—and it can provide a myriad of other health benefits. Stocking your pantry and fridge with ingredients that offer powerful nutrition benefits is the best way to create healing meals that taste good while helping your body to achieve its nutritional goals.

This chapter explores how kitchen staples such as extra-virgin olive oil, spices, beans, legumes, and whole grains, along with fresh fruits, vegetables, fish, and poultry, can transform your meals into delicious and nutritious daily experiences.

REMEMBER

The antioxidant-rich ingredients, such as extra-virgin olive oil, spices, leafy green vegetables, and so on, that we mention in this chapter are only a small sample of what you can (and should) enjoy for managing your cholesterol. In addition, wholesome whole grains such as oats, barley, and whole wheat are always good additions or substitutes for other grains.

Herbs and Spices

Several spices have known anti-inflammatory effects, which can be very beneficial for people managing their cholesterol. Anti-inflammatory ingredients in general work to prevent the oxidation of low-density lipoprotein (LDL) cholesterol, which is a key factor in the development of plaque buildup in blood vessels. Preventing the oxidation of LDL cholesterol reduces the risk of heart disease and other illnesses. In addition, all spices are "free foods," which means you can incorporate them into any meal without worrying about counting their calories, sodium, or carbohydrate.

TIP

When it comes to anti-inflammatory benefits, black pepper, cardamom, cayenne, cinnamon, cloves, garlic, ginger, saffron, and turmeric are all highly effective. You can harness the power of these flavorful ingredients by adding them to your recipes daily. You can also take a tip from the Mediterranean lifestyle and prepare them as *tisanes* (herbal teas), made by placing a teaspoon of any of these herbs and/or spices into a mug full of hot water, letting it sit for 10 minutes, straining, and drinking daily. This is a soothing and therapeutic way to start and end each day.

Chef Amy also recommends making a mouth-watering anti-inflammatory spice blend and keeping it on hand. You can use it as a rub to coat meats, fish, or poultry; sprinkle tablespoonfuls over vegetables or proteins before roasting; add it to onions and garlic while sautéing; or enjoy it steeped as a hot tisane a few times per day. Here's her recipe:

Anti-Inflammatory Spice Mix

¼ cup Ceylon ground cinnamon

¼ cup ground ginger

¼ cup ground turmeric

¼ cup ground cardamom

1 teaspoon crushed black pepper

1 teaspoon saffron threads, crushed

1 teaspoon cloves

¼ teaspoon cayenne, if desired

Place all the ingredients in a Mason jar or other large glass container, cover, and shake well to combine. Cover and store in a dark, cool place for up to a year.

TECHNICAL
STUFF

In the United States, two types of cinnamon are commonly sold: cassia cinnamon and Ceylon cinnamon. Cassia cinnamon can contain small amounts of cassia bark. Ceylon cinnamon is known as "true cinnamon" or "pure cinnamon" and has milder citrus notes. Ceylon cinnamon also contains lower levels of a compound called coumarin, which can be harmful when consumed in very large quantities. If you're using cinnamon for therapeutic properties, it's best to seek out the Ceylon variety.

Beans and Other Legumes

Beans and other legumes are nutritious, economical, and good for the environment. Culinarily speaking, they're a blank canvas on which to build flavor, and they pair well with all types of cuisines. Beans and other legumes are rich in both soluble and insoluble fiber, which work to reduce LDL cholesterol levels. They're also an important source of protein and naturally low in calories.

Black beans, cannellini beans, chickpeas, kidney beans, and others can all be prepared in batches and frozen for later use. (Chapter 13 explains how to prepare them in advance from scratch.)

TIP

If you purchase canned beans, be sure to opt for low-sodium versions or, best of all, those canned with water, and drain and rinse them well before including them in recipes.

Aim for at least ½ cup of beans and legumes per day. Try adding them to soups and salads, using them as a meat substitute in burgers, or mashing and pureeing them to make tasty dips and velvety soups.

Nuts and Seeds

A Louisiana State University study involving 13,000 subjects found that consumers of tree nuts (the study excluded peanuts) had smaller waist measurements, lower weight, lower blood pressure, lower fasting blood glucose, higher levels of high-density lipoprotein (HDL) cholesterol, and lower levels of inflammatory proteins. Regular nut eating was also linked with higher consumption of whole grains and fruits and lower consumption of alcohol and sugar. In other words, nuts are a great addition to your daily diet!

One serving of nuts contains enough protein, fiber, and fat to help you feel full. Nuts contain healthy monounsaturated and polyunsaturated fats — one ounce of nuts contains 13 to 22 grams of these heart-healthy fats. Brazil nuts, cashews, hazelnuts, peanuts (which are considered legumes), pecans, almonds, and walnuts all contain monounsaturated fats.

Nuts can help manage cholesterol by lowering LDL cholesterol and improving HDL cholesterol. Nuts are high in unsaturated fatty acids, fiber, plant stanols (see Chapter 5), and plant protein. Nuts are a great source of heart-healthy monosaturated fats and contain significant amounts of magnesium, potassium, and vitamin E.

TIP

In addition to eating 5 to 10 almonds as a snack or before meals, you can swap almond flour for white all-purpose flour in many recipes. Almond flour increases the flavor, texture, and nutritional value of many baked goods. Plus, it's a great way to make recipes gluten free and delicious! In diabetes-friendly desserts, almond flour has a special appeal because almonds contain both healthful fats and protein, which serves to balance out the natural sweeteners in the recipes.

TIP

Be sure to purchase nuts that contain no salt or sugar and that have their polyphenol-rich outer skins (see Chapter 5 for more on polyphenols). For a delicious snack that has many health benefits, try heating 1 or 2 tablespoons of good-quality extra-virgin olive oil in a large skillet. Add 1 tablespoon of the anti-inflammatory spice mix listed earlier in this chapter and 1 cup of nuts. Stir to coat and allow the nuts to sauté in the spices over medium heat until they're lightly toasted and fragrant. Serve warm or at room temperature prior to a meal. This technique will help you to eat less and absorb more nutrients from the meal.

Seeds are great for overall health management. They contain protein, fiber, and fat, which makes them filling and can help prevent the body from absorbing too much sugar, keeping glucose levels in check. And research has found that seeds can be a good replacement for carbohydrate snacks because they lower LDL cholesterol after three months.

Sesame seeds can help people with type 2 diabetes reach their target blood sugar levels. They also contain lignans and phytosterols, which are plant compounds that can help lower cholesterol.

Flaxseeds may help reduce cholesterol and triglyceride levels. They can also help people with diabetes improve blood sugar control and insulin sensitivity. Flaxseeds are rich in fiber, omega-3 fatty acids, and bioactive compounds. For more information on bioactive compounds and reducing damaging LDL cholesterol, turn to Chapter 5.

Extra-Virgin Olive Oil

Olive oil generally contains between 55 percent and 83 percent monounsaturated fat, with the rest being made up of smaller amounts of polyunsaturated and saturated fats. The main monounsaturated fat in olive oil is called *oleic acid*. Oleic acid is good for heart health, and it's the most common monounsaturated fat in the human diet. Oleic acid has been shown to lower LDL cholesterol and raise HDL cholesterol.

Because olives and olive oil are a common denominator in the countries surrounding the Mediterranean Sea, they're often analyzed in research on the Mediterranean diet. Antioxidants such as vitamin E, carotenoids, and polyphenols such as hydroxytyrosol and oleuropein (known for their anti-inflammatory and antibacterial effects) are found in olive oil.

Optimizing glucose management reduces systemic oxidation and inflammation.

Adding extra-virgin olive oil to carbohydrates has the remarkable effect of slowing their absorption as well as increasing insulin sensitivity. It also leaves your appetite more satiated sooner and your gut microbes happier. This combination results in a reduced glycemic load of a meal. Optimum blood glucose control is important to manage oxidative stress and reduce systemic inflammation, protecting LDL from damaging oxidation. (For more information, see Chapters 4 and 5.) In the recipes in this book, we use extra-virgin olive oil instead of all other oils in baking, and we even use it as a replacement for butter. Chapter 18 discusses why we like to use extra-virgin olive oil in place of butter.

TIP

For even more information on extra-virgin olive oil, check out one of our other books, *Olive Oil For Dummies* (published by Wiley).

Fish

Fish is an excellent low-fat source of protein. Salmon, swordfish, and tuna are readily available fresh and frozen and are excellent sources of not only protein, but also niacin, selenium, vitamin B6, vitamin D, and omega-3 fatty acids.

TIP

To triple the health benefits of fish when cooking it, use extra-virgin olive oil and 1 or 2 teaspoons of Chef Amy's Anti-Inflammatory Spice Mix from earlier in this chapter while roasting, broiling, sautéing, or grilling it.

TIP

If possible, choose wild salmon over farmed salmon and always check to ensure that you're enjoying sustainable types of fish. In the United States, an app produced by the Monterey Bay Aquarium (`www.seafoodwatch.org`) is continuously monitored and updated so that you can look up any type of fish and immediately find out whether it's a sustainable choice.

Whole Grains

Whole grains such as oats, barley, and 100 percent whole wheat are great sources of fiber. Fiber has long been touted by the health community as having the ability to lower LDL cholesterol. For this reason, try to combine whole grains like oatmeal and whole wheat with the other powerful ingredients in this chapter. These naturally cholesterol-free grains also help you to feel full.

Both barley and oats contain a specific soluble fiber called *beta-glucan* to help you manage cholesterol. Technically considered a carbohydrate, beta-glucan is especially effective at lowering bad LDL cholesterol levels and reducing the risk for atherosclerosis. The effectiveness of the soluble fiber in oats in impacting cholesterol levels has earned it authorization from the U.S. Food and Drug Administration (FDA) to use heart-healthy claims on product packaging.

TIP

Oats and barley aren't just for breakfast, you can also include them in soups, stews, and baking. Try swapping out oat flour or barley flour for all-purpose flour in your recipes. You can also boil barley and eat it instead of rice, or use it cold in a salad. Barley tastes great in pudding recipes, too.

Whole wheat can help reduce your LDL cholesterol and raise your HDL cholesterol. You can swap out whole-wheat flour for all-purpose flour in recipes. Try 100 percent whole-wheat pasta and bread recipes, too.

Greek Yogurt

Consuming plain, full-fat Greek yogurt as a part of a balanced diet and healthy lifestyle is important for cholesterol management. If you can eat dairy, Greek yogurt should be a staple in your refrigerator. Yogurt, especially plain Greek yogurt, is high in protein and vitamin B12, which is mostly found in animal products, making it a great protein choice for people who don't eat meat. The original Greek variety is made from a combination of goat and sheep milk, which offer additional nutrient profiles. Even cow milk has benefits; it contains a healthful dose of calcium, magnesium, potassium, vitamin B2, and vitamin B12.

Yogurt with live active cultures (called *probiotics*) is known to help maintain the natural balance of organisms, known as *microflora,* in the intestines. These beneficial bacteria may help reduce inflammation and improve gut health, which can positively impact cholesterol. The calcium content in yogurt may help block the absorption of cholesterol in the intestines.

Gut health, which we discuss in Chapter 5, is essential for well-being, especially for people trying to manage their cholesterol levels and for people with diabetes.

TIP

You can use Greek yogurt instead of sour cream and heavy cream in baking and in desserts.

Fruits and Vegetables

Fruits and vegetables contain antioxidants and bioactive compounds, which are very beneficial to health. Most of your diet should be made up of fruits and vegetables; aim for 9 to 12 servings of fresh produce per day. Consuming the adequate amount of fresh fruits and vegetables improves gut health and helps us to and harness the power of their bioactive compounds and fiber content to lower LDL cholesterol.

Fruits and vegetables that have heart-healthy, LDL-lowering effects include apples, artichokes, blueberries, citrus fruits (such as lemons, limes, and oranges), cranberries, cruciferous vegetables (such as broccoli, cabbage, and cauliflower), peas, pomegranates, raspberries, red grapes, strawberries, red cabbage, and tomatoes.

Fiber-rich apples, citrus fruits, eggplants, grapes, okra, and strawberries are also readily available additions to the diet. These fruits are rich in pectin, a type of soluble fiber that lowers LDL. All fresh fruits and vegetables offer important nutrients, but if you're interested in managing cholesterol, be sure to include these fruits and vegetables in your daily diet along with others.

TIP

Having fresh fruit with every meal is a wise choice. For this reason, we've incorporated fruit into as many of our dessert recipes as possible, in the true Mediterranean tradition. According to the Mediterranean diet, vegetables are the base of each meal and fruit itself is a daily dessert.

Chapter **18**

Ten Misconceptions about Cholesterol

As awareness of the role of cholesterol in cardiovascular disease (CVD) has increased, research has revealed new discoveries about the ways in which cholesterol affects blood vessels. Most people — including doctors — have trouble keeping up with this new knowledge. What we know for sure is that there's much more to cholesterol than the outdated simplistic belief that cholesterol blocks arteries and should be lowered with the widespread use of drugs.

In this chapter, you learn some of the most common misconceptions, many of which we explore in more detail in the relevant chapters of this book.

Myth: All Cholesterol Is Bad

Cholesterol is essential for our bodies to function properly. It plays a crucial role in building cell membranes, producing hormones like estrogen and testosterone, and helping our bodies make vitamin D. Without cholesterol, many vital processes in the body would be compromised. Problems arise when there is an imbalance in cholesterol levels, particularly an excess of low-density lipoprotein (LDL) cholesterol, especially in its most damaging, oxidized form, which can lead to plaque buildup in the arteries and increase the risk of heart disease, stroke, and other CVDs.

There are several types of circulating cholesterol, bound to proteins called *lipoproteins* (see Chapter 2). LDL, often referred to as "bad" cholesterol, and high-density lipoprotein (HDL) cholesterol, known as "good" cholesterol, are the two most important forms. High levels of LDL contributes to *arteriosclerosis* (the buildup of fatty deposits in the arteries) and CVD; HDL cholesterol helps remove excess cholesterol from the bloodstream and transport it to the liver for disposal. A healthy balance between these two types is key to maintaining good cardiovascular health.

TIP

Instead of aiming to eliminate cholesterol entirely, focus on maintaining a healthy diet, exercising regularly, and managing other risk factors to keep your cholesterol levels in check.

Myth: Cholesterol Is the Most Important Risk Factor

Cholesterol is an important risk factor for CVD, but it isn't the most significant risk factor on its own, unless it's exceptionally high, perhaps with familial hypercholesterolemia (FH). CVD is influenced by a combination of factors, including high blood pressure, smoking, diabetes, genetics, physical inactivity, and an unhealthy diet. High cholesterol, particularly elevated and oxidized LDL cholesterol, *can* contribute to arteriosclerosis, increasing the risk of heart attacks, strokes, and other cardiovascular illnesses. However, other factors, such as chronic inflammation, insulin resistance, and lifestyle choices, also play crucial roles in determining cardiovascular health.

REMEMBER

Addressing cholesterol levels is important, but it should be done as part of a broader strategy that includes maintaining a healthy weight, staying active, and managing blood pressure and blood sugar levels. All these factors are important particularly for people who have already been diagnosed with CVD. Driving down levels of LDL cholesterol for these people is even more important, and this is often done with medications like statins.

Myth: Only Overweight People Have High Cholesterol

Another common misconception is that only overweight people have high cholesterol. Excess body weight *can* contribute to unhealthy cholesterol levels, but many lean or normal-weight individuals can also have high cholesterol due to genetics, diet, or other metabolic factors. FH, for example, is an inherited condition that leads to high cholesterol levels regardless of body weight. Additionally, diets high in saturated and trans fats, lack of physical activity, and even certain medical conditions like *hypothyroidism* (an underactive thyroid gland can cause cholesterol levels to rise) can cause high cholesterol. Other hormonal influences on cholesterol may come into play when a person is suffering from chronic stress, poor sleep, or other less tangible negative effects on well-being and mental health.

REMEMBER

Because cholesterol levels are influenced by multiple factors beyond weight alone, regular checkups and blood tests are essential for assessing cardiovascular risk and maintaining heart health.

Myth: Cholesterol Simply Blocks Arteries

The idea that too much cholesterol simply "clogs" arteries over time, much like grease building up in a pipe, is an oversimplification of a much more complex process. High levels of LDL cholesterol *can* contribute to the formation of arterial plaques, but the real danger lies in how these plaques behave rather than just their presence. Arteriosclerosis is not just about cholesterol accumulating in the blood vessels — it's driven by a combination of oxidative stress, inflammation, and immune system responses (see Chapter 4).

When LDL cholesterol particles become oxidized, they trigger an inflammatory reaction in the artery walls. The body responds by sending white blood cells to absorb the oxidized LDL, forming foam cells that contribute to plaque formation. However, not all plaques are equally dangerous; some remain stable and cause only mild narrowing, while others are more vulnerable to rupture. If a plaque breaks apart, it can lead to the formation of a blood clot that may suddenly block an artery, causing a heart attack, stroke, or critical loss of blood supply to another vital organ. Systemic inflammation, poor metabolic health, and lifestyle factors such as smoking, a poor diet, and chronic stress all can influence plaque stability and increase cardiovascular risk. Understanding this broader picture highlights the importance of not only managing cholesterol levels but also reducing inflammation and oxidative stress through the lifestyle approaches described in this book.

Myth: Everything That Matters Is Measured in Risk Calculator Tools

CVD risk calculators are useful tools for estimating the likelihood of developing heart disease or stroke based on well-established factors such as cholesterol levels, blood pressure, smoking status, and diabetes. Doctors commonly use them to inform decisions about whether to recommend cholesterol-lowering medications to people without symptoms with a ten-year risk of CVD above particular thresholds. These models *are* valuable for assessing average risk across populations, but they have limitations when it comes to evaluating an individual's true risk. One major shortcoming is that they don't directly measure key biological processes like oxidative stress, systemic and local inflammation, or plaque stability, factors that play a critical role in whether atherosclerosis leads to serious events like heart attacks or strokes.

For example, two people with similar cholesterol levels may have very different risks depending on how much of their LDL cholesterol is oxidized or whether they have high levels of inflammatory markers like high sensitivity C-reactive protein (HS-CRP). Similarly, someone with relatively mild arterial plaque buildup may be at greater risk than someone with more extensive plaques if their plaques are unstable and prone to rupture. These factors are often influenced by lifestyle choices.

Because most risk calculators rely on broad, easily measurable factors, they can sometimes overestimate risk in some individuals and underestimate it in others. This emphasizes the importance of the more personalized approach to cholesterol management and cardiovascular health described throughout this book that goes beyond standard risk scores to consider lifestyle and metabolic health, and looks forward to when advanced biomarkers that offer a deeper understanding of an individual's true risk profile are more widely available.

Myth: Success Is Measured by a Lipid Panel

The fact that oxidation of LDL cholesterol and chronic inflammation, locally in arteriosclerotic plaques or more systemically, are not yet measured as part of routine cholesterol management means that doctors and patients deal simply with the numbers provided by the lipid panel and CVD risk calculators.

REMEMBER

If you take a positive approach to your cholesterol levels through lifestyle measures such as having an improved diet, getting more regular exercise, and reducing the effects of chronic stress, you'll reap significant rewards. The effects on your lipid panel results (as well as your blood pressure and body mass index, or BMI) may be great or perhaps disappointingly small. Of the limited measurements entered into the algorithm, your age has much more influence on your CVD risk calculation than your lipid panel result, so you may not even see a big change in your calculated risk even if your LDL cholesterol does reduce. However, the benefits to your physical and mental well-being of a healthy lifestyle will be profound. Plus, although they're not easily measured and perhaps not a topic of conversation in the doctor's office, your oxidized LDL and background chronic inflammation — and thus, your real risk of CVD — will be reduced. Effective cholesterol management is about much more than just reducing measurable numbers.

Myth: You Can't Lower Cholesterol Risk without Medications

According to a study published in 2023 analyzing data from the Medical Expenditure Panel Survey (MEPS), the number of individuals in the general U.S. population who reported taking a statin increased from 31 million (12 percent) in 2008–2009 to 92 million (35 percent) in 2018–2019, representing a 197 percent increase. This substantial growth is largely attributed to the adoption of the 2013 American College of Cardiology (ACC) and American Heart Association (AHA) guidelines, which expanded the criteria for statin eligibility.

These statistics show how frequently statins are prescribed to reduce cholesterol. Although most guidelines recommend changes to diet and increasing exercise as a first step, doctors often place little emphasis on targeted improvements in lifestyle factors. Medications may be (incorrectly) considered to be the quickest and simplest way to meet a target to lower cholesterol.

Lifestyle changes can have a significant effect on cholesterol levels, reducing harmful LDL cholesterol and increasing beneficial HDL cholesterol, thus reducing the overall cholesterol ratio (see Chapters 9 and 10).

REMEMBER

It's not just a numbers game. It's even more important to lessen the *risks associated* with high cholesterol, as well as the simple measured results. Positive lifestyle changes will not only decrease LDL cholesterol and the cholesterol ratio, but also reduce harmful oxidative stress and chronic inflammation, which are known to increase the risks of a person with any given cholesterol level ending up with arteriosclerosis, heart attack, or stroke.

Myth: I Can Eat Whatever I Want Because I Take a Statin

A common misconception is that drug treatment for high cholesterol cures the problem and solves the issue of any increased risk of arteriosclerosis. A person may even believe that forgetting to take their medication for a few days may immediately put them at risk of having a heart attack or stroke. The reality is not quite as straightforward.

Taking medications like statins has an effect over time, and outcomes are not guaranteed or certain. Depending on factors such as age and overall risk, taking a medication may lessen the chances of having a heart attack or stroke by 20 percent to 30 percent in an otherwise healthy person without established heart disease or other vascular symptoms. However, many people taking a medication wouldn't have had a heart attack or stroke even if they weren't taking that medication. Others may take a medication conscientiously every day, perhaps putting up with side effects, and go on to have a heart attack or stroke anyway. Some people may be taking medications that prevent a heart attack or stroke, but they won't know when and where this event would've taken place.

TIP

Plenty of research shows that taking cholesterol-lowering medication is very effective in preventing further events such as a heart attacks or strokes for people who've already been diagnosed with heart or other vascular diseases. The risk of a further event is much higher, and the reduction in risk achieved with medication is more likely to be greater as well (for example, 30 percent to 40 percent, depending on various factors). Medications like statins, alongside lifestyle changes, are key to secondary prevention of CVD and are routinely recommended by healthcare professionals.

REMEMBER

Taking medications like statins may be an important step in secondary prevention of CVD, and they're frequently considered for primary prevention. However, their use doesn't mean that you can safely eat a poor diet or have a sedentary lifestyle even with a reduced cholesterol. If you're thought to have a high risk of heart attack or stroke and offered a drug that lowers your cholesterol, it's even *more* important to enjoy an excellent healthy diet and get plenty of exercise to further minimize that risk.

Myth: A Low-Fat Diet Is Best

For many years, people were encouraged to eat a low-fat diet as a way to manage cholesterol and reduce the risk of heart disease. However, we now know that this advice is overly simplistic and, in some cases, even misleading. Not all fats are harmful. Healthy fats found in extra-virgin olive oil, nuts, seeds, and oily fish can actually *improve* cholesterol levels by raising HDL, the "good" cholesterol, and supporting overall cardiovascular health with the other nutrients these foods contain. Many low-fat products are highly processed, containing sugar and other unhealthy ingredients.

REMEMBER

One of the best dietary patterns for cholesterol management is the Mediterranean diet, which emphasizes these healthy fats alongside fresh vegetables, whole grains, legumes, and lean proteins like fish. This diet, and other heritage or traditional diets, are not only effective in lowering LDL cholesterol but also help reduce inflammation and oxidative stress, improve blood vessel function, and support overall metabolic health. A key component of this approach is a diet's richness in *polyphenols,* naturally occurring plant compounds found in foods like berries, coffee, dark chocolate, extra-virgin olive oil, and colorful vegetables and fruits. Polyphenols have been shown to reduce oxidative stress, enhance HDL function, and promote plaque stability, all of which contribute to better cardiovascular outcomes.

TIP

Instead of focusing simply on cutting out fat, a better approach is to prioritize whole, nutrient-dense foods and include heart-healthy fats as part of a balanced, sustainable Mediterranean diet.

Myth: Sugar Has No Effect on Cholesterol

Another common incorrect notion is that sugar has no impact on cholesterol levels. Sugar doesn't contain cholesterol, but consuming too much added sugar can contribute to unhealthy cholesterol and triglyceride levels.

Diets high in refined carbohydrates and added sugars can lead to insulin resistance, increased fat production in the liver, and higher levels of small, dense LDL particles — the type most associated with CVD. Excess sugar intake also promotes systemic inflammation, which plays a key role in the progression of arteriosclerosis toward heart disease and stroke. High sugar consumption can also contribute to *nonalcoholic fatty liver disease* (NAFLD), a condition in which fat accumulates in the liver, impairing its ability to regulate cholesterol and triglyceride levels.

Eating too many sugar-sweetened beverages, processed snacks, and refined grains is now recognized as a major driver of *metabolic syndrome* — a cluster of conditions that includes high blood pressure, abdominal obesity, and abnormal cholesterol levels. This is why reducing added sugars, particularly from sugary drinks and processed foods, is just as important for cholesterol management as moderating unhealthy fats. A diet rich in fiber, healthy fats, and minimally processed foods not only supports better cholesterol balance but also helps prevent insulin resistance and inflammation, two key drivers of CVD.

Index

A

absolute risk, 110, 119

acromegaly, 36

acupressure, 169

acupuncture, 168–169

acute inflammation, 52. *See also* inflammation

acute pancreatitis, 26

acute phase response, 24

addictions, 125

adrenaline, 34–35, 137

aerobic exercise, 32. *See also* exercise

age, 22–23, 37, 41, 112–113

age-related macular degeneration, 12

air pollution, 35, 49

alcohol

  cholesterol in, 65

  high cholesterol and, 34

  inflammation and, 53

  limiting, 209

  oxidative stress and, 49

  as risk factor, 125

algorithms, 101, 105, 106–107, 111–114

alirocumab, 158

almond flour, 262

Amy Riolo Selections Extra Virgin Olive Oil, 214

aneurysm, 45–46

angina, 54, 150

angiography, 46

angiotensin-converting enzyme (ACE), 163

Anichkov, Nikolai, 11

anthocyanins, 92

Anti-Inflammatory Spice Mix recipe, 260

antioxidants, 42, 74, 177–179

anxiety, 117

APOB gene, 30–31

apolipoprotein B (ApoB), 120

Apolipoprotein B (ApoB) test, 27

appetitive naps, 129

appetizers, recipes for, 221–227

Apple Cinnamon Oatmeal with Toasted Almonds recipe, 216

arcus corneae, 31

arteries, 9, 269–270

arterioles, 9

arteriosclerosis, 9, 11, 40. *See also* heart disease

Artichoke, Pea, and Cherry Tomato Salad with Lemon and Basil Dressing recipe, 237

artificial sweeteners, 66, 67

atherosclerosis, 9, 10, 39–40, 45, 212

Atherosclerotic Cardiovascular Disease (ASCVD) Risk Estimator, 105–106

ATP-citrate lyase (ACL) inhibitors, 156

autoimmune illnesses, 35, 152

autosomal dominant, 31

Avocado, Citrus, and Spinach Salad with Walnuts and White Balsamic Vinaigrette recipe, 240

B

Baby Artichokes recipe, 190

barley, 264

Barley and Red Wine "Risotto" with Red Cabbage and Cannellini Beans recipe, 233

beans, 178, 186, 188, 197–198, 261

bempedoic acid, 156

berberine, 170

bergamot, 170

betablockers, 35

beta-glucan, 72, 264

bile acid sequestrants, 155

bile acids, 18, 72, 151, 155

bioactive compounds, 75, 81

biomarkers, 93, 113

blood clot (thrombus), 44, 45, 57, 103, 269

blood pressure, 121, 124

blood tests
  categorization of levels of cholesterol in, 23–24
  function of, 47
  ordering of, 8
  process of, 22
  public opinion regarding, 14
  statistics regarding, 7
blood vessels, 9, 12, 41, 55, 139
blood-brain barrier, 19
body mass index (BMI), 84–85, 105, 113
brain, 19
bread, 66
breakfast, recipes for, 214–220
breathwork, 141–142
butter, 64
butylated hydroxyanisole (BHA), 66
butylated hydroxytoluene (BHT), 66
bypass surgery, 162

C

calcium, 75
Calm, 124
calories, 84–85
Cannellini Beans recipe, 188
capillaries, 9, 45
capric acid, 64
caprylic acid, 64
carbohydrate metabolism, 10
carbohydrates
  cholesterol regulation and, 61–62
  complex, 87
  in diet comparisons, 82
  extra-virgin olive oil and, 263
  myth regarding, 273–274
  oxidative stress and inflammation and, 67
  refined, 65, 71
cardiovascular diseases (CVDs). *See also* vascular
    diseases; *specific diseases*
  causes of, 13
  checking risks for, 257
  costs of, 12, 83

death from, 12
harm to the body by, 11–13
inflammation and, 13, 29
oxidation and, 13, 29
primary prevention of, 14, 99–103, 116, 152–153, 158, 159
secondary prevention of, 14, 100, 109, 151, 152, 158, 159
statistics regarding, 12
symptoms of, 150
carotenoids, 75
carotid artery, 86
carotid endarterectomy, 163
cells, 18, 49
Centers for Disease Control and Prevention (CDC), 7
cerebrovascular accident (stroke), 12, 43, 55–56, 162
cerebrovascular disease, 11
Ceylon cinnamon, 261
chakras, 171
chickpeas, 187
Chocolate Ginger Waffles with Vanilla Berry Syrup recipe, 220
cholesterol
  calculating risk of, 99–107
  categorization of levels of, 23–24
  circulating, 61
  complexity of, 10
  complications regarding, 10
  function of, 17, 267–268
  history of the study of, 11
  importance of, 17–20
  integrated approach to, 13–16
  as leading to chronic disease, 45–46
  lipid theory of, 40–47
  management of, 44–45
  manufacturing of, 18
  measuring, 21–25
  measuring effects of, 46–47
  misconceptions of, 267–274
  misunderstandings of, 8
  personal meaning of, 8

purpose of, 160

regulation of, 18

as risk factor, 268–269

role of, 18–19, 267–268

as sterol, 18, 73, 157

structure of, 18

types of, 19–20 (*see also specific types*)

cholesterol absorption inhibitors, 154

Cholesterol and Recurrent Events (CARE), 151

cholesterol oxidation, 10

cholesterol ratio, 22, 25

Cholesterol Trialists' Collaboration (CTT), 104

cholestyramine, 155

chronic inflammation, 10, 36, 52. *See also* inflammation

chronic kidney disease (CKD), 33–34, 152

chronic liver disease, 33–34

chronic stress. *See* stress/chronic stress

chylomicrons, 20, 26

cinnamon, 261

circulating cholesterol, 61, 101

Classic Hummus with Crudites recipe, 227

claudication, 150

coagulation cascade, 44

coffee, 92

cognition, 56

colesevelam, 155

collateral vessels, 46

community-supported agriculture (CSA), 176

comorbidities, 160

complementary therapies, 167–172

computed tomography (CT) scan, 46

confounding factors, 69–70

connection, social, 129–131

continuous glucose monitors (CGMs), 121

cooking. *See also* diet; foods

  with antioxidant-rich foods, 177–179

  finding time for, 199–201

  making whole foods taste great in, 180–182

  meal planning for, 176–177

  overview of, 175

  preparing base recipes for, 182–193

  shortcuts in, 200

cooking oils, 68

CORDIOPREV study, 86

cornea, 31

coronary artery bypass grafting (CABG) (bypass surgery), 162

coronary artery calcium (CAC) scan, 120

coronary heart disease (heart disease), 11. *See also* heart disease

cortisol, 18, 34–35, 126–127, 130, 137

C-reactive protein (CRP), 53, 135

culinary medicine, 15–16

Cushing's disease, 36

D

dairy, 70–71, 81, 90–91

dark chocolate, 71, 92

death, 12, 63

Decadent Dark Chocolate Mousse with Strawberries recipe, 246

decorating, kitchen, 197

dessert recipes, 241–248

diabetes, 10, 13, 33, 56–57, 83, 152

diabetic dyslipidemia, 33

diabetic retinopathy, 12

diet. *See also* cooking; foods; Mediterranean diet/lifestyle

  anti-inflammatory, 53

  benefits of, 133

  characteristics of, 79–80

  CVD and vascular diseases and, 13

  excess salt in, 68

  foods that raise cholesterol in, 62–71

  heritage, 95, 221, 228

  high cholesterol and, 32

  inflammation and, 53

  myth regarding, 273

  overview of, 61–62

  oxidative stress and, 49

  reactive oxygen species (ROS) and, 51

  as risk factor, 124

  sleep and, 127

  Western, 72-73, 82–85, 94

dining out, 208–209, 255

Direct LDL-C test, 27

dizziness, 150

dopamine, 143, 144

Doppler ultrasound, 46

Dried Beans recipe, 186

Dried Chickpeas recipe, 187

dyslipidemia, 66, 87, 130

E

eating out, 208–209, 255

elastin, 41

elderly, statins and, 117

electrocardiograms (EKGs), 47

emboli, 54

Emotional Freedom Technique (EFT), 169

emotional well-being, 166–167

endorphins, 143, 144

endothelial function, 139

endothelial function tests, 120

endothelium, 41, 43, 68

environmental pollution, 53

EPIC study, 89

epidemics, 200

essential naps, 129

estrogen, 18, 37

ethnicity, as risk factor, 114

European Atherosclerosis Society (EAS), 23

European Food Safety Authority (EFSA), 89–90

European Society of Cardiology (ESC), 23, 102, 106, 158

evolocumab, 158

exercise

benefits of, 124, 133, 134–136

choosing, 136

enjoying, 255–256

hobbies as, 136

inflammation and, 135

in Mediterranean diet, 81, 136

plaque stability and, 135

reactive oxygen species (ROS) and, 51

resistance training as, 136

resources for, 137

risk reduction from, 112, 114

sleep and, 128

stress and, 138

extra-virgin olive oil

benefits of, 212, 252

choosing, 213–214

components of, 88

embracing, 254

importance of, 179–180

with nuts, 262

oleic acid in, 178

overview of, 263

special role of, 89–90

eyes, 12, 56

ezetimibe, 151, 154

F

familial combined hyperlipidemia (FCHL), 30

familial hypercholesterolemia (FH), 30–31, 152, 269

family history, 113

fasting, intermittent, 215

fats. See also extra-virgin olive oil

avoiding unhealthy, 179

chemistry of, 63–64

in diet comparisons, 82

healthy, 73, 213, 252, 273

in Mediterranean diet, 84–85

monounsaturated, 63, 64, 73

polyunsaturated, 63, 64, 73

saturated, 32, 63–64, 69–70, 252

stanols, 73

trans, 32, 62–63, 179, 252

unsaturated, 32, 63, 73

fenofibrate, 155

fiber, 71–73, 213, 251–252, 264

fibrates, 155

fish, 88, 178, 263–264

fish oil, 170

flavonoids, 71, 91–92

flaxseeds, 170, 262

flushing, 155

foam cells, 43

focused meditation, 143

Food and Drug Administration (FDA), 72, 89, 264

foods. *See also* cooking; diet; *specific foods*
anti-inflammatory, 212, 260
antioxidant-rich, 177–179, 259–265
bioactive compounds in, 75, 81
cholesterol in, 65
cholesterol-friendly, 71–77, 212–213, 259–265
for eating out, 208–209, 255
fiber-rich, 71–73, 252
finding time for cooking, 199–201
at high temperatures, 67–68
inflammation and, 67
labels, 68–69, 253
for lowering cholesterol, 87–91
macronutrients in, 74, 81
making list of appropriate, 201
meal planning of, 176–177, 201–208, 255
micronutrients in, 74, 81
myth regarding, 272
oxidative stress and, 67, 75–76
polyphenols in, 75–76, 77, 91
portion sizes for, 201, 209
processed, 65–66
pro-inflammatory, 67
protein in, 74
reading labels of, 68–69, 253
seven-day meal plan, 203–208
ultra-processed, 32, 62, 66–67, 200
vitamins and minerals in, 74–75
whole, 70–71

4S Study (Scandinavian Simvastatin Survival Study), 14, 151

Framingham Heart Study, 11, 40, 107

Framingham Risk Score, 107

free radicals, 20, 41–42, 48, 49–50, 51, 135

freezer, 198–199, 202

French paradox, 69–70

Fresh Breadcrumbs recipe, 193

Fresh Summer Berry Clafoutis recipe, 247

fruits, 88, 92, 177–179, 265

fulfillment naps, 129

full lipid panel/profile, 8

G

gemfibrozil, 155

gender, as risk factor, 112–113

gene therapy, 161

genetics, 30–31, 49, 112–113, 257

goat dairy, 70–71

Greek yogurt, 178, 264–265

Greek Yogurt with Honey, Pomegranate, and Avocado Parfait recipe, 218

green tea, 170

guided imagery meditation, 142

gut microbiome, 65–66, 72, 76–77

H

happiness, 140, 143–144, 167, 171

Haslam, David, 116

HDL cholesterol (HDL-C) component, 21, 22, 24, 33. *See also* cholesterol; *specific effects*

Headspace, 124, 142

heart age, 111

heart attack, 12, 43, 54–55, 110

heart disease, 9–10, 11, 12, 110. *See also* arteriosclerosis; cardiovascular diseases (CVDs); *specific diseases*

heart failure, 54

Herb Roasted Fish with Vegetables and Brown Rice Pilaf recipe, 229–230

herbal teas, 260

herbs and spices, 92, 178–179, 181, 198, 260–261

heritage diets, 95, 221, 228

high blood glucose, 56–57

high blood pressure, 11, 13, 68, 126

high cholesterol
  age factor for, 22–23
  air pollution and, 35
  alcohol and, 34
  as asymptomatic, 31
  categories of, 30
  causes of, 31–37
  chronic inflammation and, 36
  chronic kidney or liver disease and,
    33–34
  chronic stress and, 34–35
  diet and, 32
  diseases from, 53–57
  factors of, 30
  familial, 30–31
  hormones and, 35–36
  inflammation and, 29
  life stages and, 37
  mental health and, 171
  misunderstandings of, 8
  obesity and, 33
  overview of, 29
  oxidation and, 29
  sleep and, 34–35
  smoking and, 35
  statistics regarding, 7, 211
  type 2 diabetes and, 33
high-density lipoprotein (HDL). *See also*
    cholesterol; *specific effects*
  as circulating cholesterol, 101
  exercise and, 124, 134
  functionality, 48
  high blood glucose and, 57
  overview of, 19–20
  oxidation and, 48
  stress and, 138
  variability in, 25
HMG-CoA reductase, 102, 154
holistic approaches, 165–167
Homemade Chicken Stock recipe, 185
Homemade Vegetable Stock recipe, 184

hormones
  cholesterol and, 18
  defined, 18, 35
  happiness, 143–144
  high cholesterol and, 35–36
  sleep and, 126, 128
  stress and, 256
hs-CRP, 107
hydrogenation, 32
hypercholesterolemia, 18, 101
hyperthyroidism, 36
hypothalamic-pituitary-adrenal (HPA) axis, 130
hypothyroidism, 36, 269

I

ice cream, 71
icosapent ethyl (Vascepa), 157
Ikaria, 87
ILERVAS cohort study, 86
immune response, 43
in vitro investigations, 91
in vivo investigations, 91
Indian Ayurvedic tradition, 215
individual risk, 109, 110–114
Individual Spiced Apple Pies with Almond and
    Oatmeal Crust recipe, 242–243
industrialization, 200
infarction, 55
inflammation
  in cardiovascular diseases (CVDs), 13, 29
  causes of, 53
  cholesterol-friendly foods for reducing, 212
  exercise and, 135
  foods and, 67
  kidney disease and, 34
  Mediterranean diet and, 91–94
  melatonin and, 126
  obesity and, 33
  overview of, 47, 51–53
  reducing, 91–94, 135
  risk assessment tools for, 120

self-care for, 124

social connection and, 130

statins and, 102–103

stress and, 139

type 2 diabetes and, 57

inflammatory autoimmune conditions, 152

inflammatory bowel disease (IBD), 36

inflammatory markers, 53

insoluble fiber, 72

insulin, 32, 121

insulin resistance, 32, 126

integrative medicine, 166

InterHeart Risk Score, 107

intermediate-density lipoprotein (IDL), 20

intermittent fasting, 215

inventory, kitchen, 196

ischemia, 41, 46, 54

ischemic heart disease, 41, 54

isolation, 130

Italian Barley, Bean, and Mixed Vegetable Soup recipe, 224

Italian Grape Harvest Cake with Cinnamon-Red Wine Reduction recipe, 244–245

Italian Pasta with Creamy Lentils and Pecorino Cheese recipe, 234

K

Keys, Ancel, 40, 85

kidneys, 12, 56, 117

kitchen, 195–199, 200. *See also* cooking; foods

L

lauric acid, 64

law enforcement, stress and, 138

LDL-C (LDL cholesterol) component, 21, 22, 23, 33. *See also* cholesterol; specific effects

legumes, 88, 197–198, 261

lentils, 178, 189

Lentils recipe, 189

life expectancy, 83

lifestyle, 15–16, 114–115, 144–145, 166, 271. *See also* Mediterranean diet/lifestyle; specific aspects

lifestyle medicine, 15, 112

limb ischemia, 150

limbs, blood supply damage to, 12

lipid panel test, 21, 22–25, 270–271

lipid theory of cholesterol, 40–47, 69–70

lipids, 10, 11, 18, 24–25, 41

lipoprotein(a) (Lp(a)), 120

lipoproteins, 20, 268

liver

blood supply damage to, 12

cholesterol production in, 18, 34

chronic liver disease, 33–34

HMG-CoA reductase and, 102

nonalcoholic fatty liver disease (NAFLD) and, 273

statins and, 117

very low-density lipoprotein (VLDL-C) component and, 33

Lobstein, Jean, 11

lomitapide, 156

loneliness, 130

Long-term Intervention with Pravastatin in Ischemic Heart Disease (LIPID) trials, 151

loving-kindness meditation, 143

low-density lipoprotein (LDL). *See also* cholesterol; *specific effects*

as circulating cholesterol, 101

excess, 41

exercise and, 124, 134

goal levels of, 158

high blood glucose and, 57

how low is too low in, 159–160

inflammation and, 52

measuring, 48–49

obesity and, 33

overview of, 19

oxidation of, 20, 40, 41–42, 44, 48–49, 52–53, 134–135, 269

statins for, 151

stress and, 138, 139

targets of, 159

variability in, 25

lungs, blood supply damage to, 12

lupus, 152

M

macronutrients, 74, 81

macrophages, 43

macrovascular system, 9, 45

magnesium, 75, 127–128

magnetic resonance imaging (MRI) scan, 46

main courses recipes, 228–234

mantra meditation, 143

Marinated Salmon and Brussels Sprouts over Citrus Cream Sauce recipe, 231

mature atherosclerotic plaque, 43

meal planning, 176–177, 201–208, 255

meats, in Western diet, 94. *See also* protein

mechanical thrombectomy, 162

Medical Expenditure Panel Survey (MEPS), 271

medical model of care, 15, 112

medications, cholesterol-lowering. *See also specific medications*

  benefits of, 272

  complementary therapies with, 167–172

  consideration of, 150–153

  drug interactions in, 160

  false sense of security from, 13

  future research and developments in, 161

  monitoring, 161

  myth regarding, 271–272

  overtreatment with, 116

  personalizing, 157–161

  in primary prevention of CVD, 14

  risk of, 116

  as secondary prevention, 150–152

  surveying, 153–157

  targets and dosing in, 158–159

  value of, 7

MEDIMACS trial, 86

meditation, 124, 138, 142–143

Mediterranean diet/lifestyle

  affordability of, 94

  antioxidants in, 177–179

  benefits of, 77, 253–254, 273

  body mass index (BMI) and, 84–85

  defining, 80–82

  exercise and, 81, 136

  extra-virgin olive oil in, 89–90

  fats and calories in, 84–85

  focus on, 253–254

  herbal teas in, 260

  lower risk of health conditions and, 85

  making it work for you, 87–95

  overview of, 80–82

  PREDIMED Study for, 85–86

  recommendations of, 221

  reducing oxidative stress and inflammation in, 91–94

  risk reduction from, 112, 114

  social connection in, 129–131

  sustainability of, 94

  weighing evidence for, 85–87

  Western diet as compared to, 82–85

medium-chain fatty acids (MCFAs), 70–71

melatonin, 126

menopause, 37

mental health, 114, 130, 171

mesenteric artery, 56

metabolic health, 121

metabolic syndrome, 26, 274

metabolism, 33

metaphysical healing, 170–172

microbiota, 178

microflora, 265

micronutrients, 74, 81

microsomal triglyceride transfer protein (MTP) inhibitors, 156

microvascular system, 9, 45

mind-body therapy, 168, 172

mindfulness, 124, 138, 142–143

mindfulness meditation, 142

minerals, 74–75

monocytes, 43

monounsaturated fats, 63, 64, 73

Monterey Bay Aquarium, 264

Moroccan Carrot Salad recipe, 239

movement meditation, 142

myelin, 19

myocardial infarction (heart attack), 12, 43, 54–55, 110

myristic acid, 64

N

napping, 128–129. *See also* sleep

National Cholesterol Education Program (NCEP), 23

National Institute for Health and Care Excellence (NICE), 102, 116, 158, 159

National Sleep Foundation (NSF), 128

necrosis, 43

necrotic cells, 43

needed to harm (NNH), 119

needed to treat (NNT), 119

neurotransmitters, 19

niacin (vitamin B3), 74, 155

nitrates, 163

NMR LipoProfile test, 27

nonalcoholic fatty liver disease (NAFLD), 273

non-HDL cholesterol, 21, 24

nutrition labels, 68–69, 253

nuts, 88, 178, 197, 261–262

O

oats, 264

obesity

  cholesterol myth regarding, 269

  CVD and vascular diseases and, 13

  in diet comparisons, 83

  high cholesterol and, 33

  inflammation and, 53

  as risk factor, 10, 113

oleic acid, 178, 179–180

olive oil, 81, 84, 88, 89–90, 263. *See also* extra-virgin olive oil

omega fatty acids, 73, 157

Orange and Olive Oil Walnut Cake recipe, 248

organosulfur compounds, 75

overtreatment, risk of, 116

overweight, cholesterol myth regarding, 269

oxidation

  in cardiovascular diseases (CVDs), 13, 29

  defined, 11, 20, 41

  exercise and, 134–135

  of high-density lipoprotein (HDL), 48

  importance of, 40

  of low-density lipoprotein (LDL), 20, 40, 41–42, 44, 48–49, 52–53, 134–135, 269

  measuring, 48–49

  overview of, 47

  process of, 41–42, 48–49

  statins and, 103

oxidative stress

  defined, 10, 35, 42

  foods and, 67, 75–76

  Mediterranean diet and, 91–94

  melatonin and, 126

  overview of, 49–51

  polyphenols and, 75–76

  psychological stress and, 139

  reducing, 91–94

oxytocin, 143, 144

P

palliative care, 117

palmitic acid, 64

palpitations, 150

pantry, stocking, 197–198

PCSK9 gene, 31

PCSK9 inhibitors, 156, 158

pectin, 66, 265

percutaneous coronary intervention (PCI) (angioplasty) 162

peripheral artery disease (PAD), 12, 150, 162–163

peripheral vascular disease, 56

phagocytosis, 43

physical inactivity, 10, 13, 32, 124

phytosterols, 73

pita chips, 181, 191

plaque(s)
  atherosclerotic, 44
  blood clots and, 269
  cholesterol oxidation and, 10
  defined, 9
  exercise and, 135
  formation of, 41, 43, 44
  history of the study of, 11
  illustration of, 9
  instability and rupture, 43–46, 54
  stable, 43
  statins and, 103
platelets, 54
polycystic ovary syndrome (PCOS), 36
polygenic, 30
polygenic hypercholesterolemia, 30
polyphenols, 34, 75–76, 77, 91, 212, 254, 273
polyunsaturated fats, 63, 73
Pomegranate and Walnut Dip with Za'atar Spiced
  Pita Chips recipe, 222
Pooled Cohort Equations, 107
portion sizes for, 201
poultry, 90
prebiotics, 77
PREDIMED Study, 85–86, 89
pregnancy, 37
preparation, meal, 202–203
primary prevention, 14, 99–103, 116, 152–
  153, 158, 159
probiotics, 77, 178, 265
Proceedings of the National Academy of Sciences
  (journal), 129
processed foods, 65–66. *See also* foods
progressive relaxation meditation, 143
pro-inflammatory foods, 67
proinflammatory state, 53
prophylactic naps, 128
Prospective Urban Rural Epidemiology (PURE)
  study, 69–70
protein, 74, 82, 198
psoriasis, 152
publication bias, 104
pulmonary embolism, 12

pulmonary hypertension, 12
pulse wave velocity (PWV), 47

Q

QRISK Risk Calculator, 105, 106, 111

R

race, as risk factor, 114
radiation, 50
randomized controlled trials (RCTs), 104
ratio calculations, 21
reactive oxygen species (ROS), 35,
  41–42, 49–50, 51
recipes
  Anti-Inflammatory Spice Mix, 260
  appetizer, 221–227
  Apple Cinnamon Oatmeal with Toasted
    Almonds, 216
  Artichoke, Pea, and Cherry Tomato Salad with
    Lemon and Basil Dressing, 237
  Avocado, Citrus, and Spinach Salad with Walnuts
    and White Balsamic Vinaigrette, 240
  Barley and Red Wine "Risotto" with Red Cabbage
    and Cannellini Beans, 233
  for breakfast, 214–220
  Chocolate Ginger Waffles with Vanilla Berry
    Syrup, 220
  Classic Hummus with Crudites, 227
  Decadent Dark Chocolate Mousse with
    Strawberries, 246
  dessert, 241–248
  Fresh Summer Berry Clafoutis, 247
  Greek Yogurt with Honey, Pomegranate, and
    Avocado Parfait, 218
  Herb Roasted Fish with Vegetables and Brown
    Rice Pilaf, 229–230
  Individual Spiced Apple Pies with Almond and
    Oatmeal Crust, 242–243
  Italian Barley, Bean, and Mixed
    Vegetable Soup, 224
  Italian Grape Harvest Cake with Cinnamon-Red
    Wine Reduction, 244–245
  Italian Pasta with Creamy Lentils and Pecorino
    Cheese, 234

main course, 228–234

Marinated Salmon and Brussels Sprouts over Citrus Cream Sauce, 231

Moroccan Carrot Salad, 239

Orange and Olive Oil Walnut Cake, 248

overview of, 211

Pomegranate and Walnut Dip with Za'atar Spiced Pita Chips, 222

Red Berry, Dark Chocolate, and Chia Seed Overnight Pudding, 217

Red Cabbage, Citrus, and Carrot Slaw with Cilantro Vinaigrette, 236

Red Lentil "Meatballs" with Tomato Basil Sauce, 225–226

salad, 235–240

small plate, 221–227

Spiced Quinoa and Lentil Sliders, 223

Spinach, Lentil, and Pomegranate Salad, 238

Sweet Cardamom-Scented Barley and Strawberry Pudding with Nuts, 219

Vegetable Stir-Fry with Edamame and Brown Rice Noodles, 232

recovery naps, 128

Red Berry, Dark Chocolate, and Chia Seed Overnight Pudding recipe, 217

Red Cabbage, Citrus, and Carrot Slaw with Cilantro Vinaigrette recipe, 236

Red Lentil "Meatballs" with Tomato Basil Sauce recipe, 225–226

red wine, 91

redox system, 49, 51

reduction, 49

refrigerator, stocking, 199

reiki, 169

relative risk, 110

restaurants, 208–209

Reynolds Risk Score, 107

rhabdomyolysis, 154

rheumatoid arthritis, 36, 152

risk assessment tools. See also specific tools

  function of, 105

  of the future, 120–121

  inflammation and, 120

limitations of, 111–114, 161, 270

myth regarding, 270

overview of, 105–106

risk/risk factors

  absolute, 110, 119

  alcohol as, 125

  biomarkers for, 113

  of cholesterol, 99–107

  compensation, 13

  diet as, 124

  exercise and, 134–136

  interpreting, 110–114

  lowering, 271

  management, 13–15

  physical inactivity as, 124

  in primary prevention, 101–102

  relative, 110

  score, interpreting, 110–111

  sleep and, 126–129

  smoking as, 124

  social connection and, 129–131

  stress and, 137–145

  stress as, 125

  substance use disorder as, 124

  treating for reduction of, 102–103

  variation of, 270

Roasted Red Peppers recipe, 192

Ross, Russell, 11

S

salad recipes, 235–240

salmon, 264

salt, 68, 181–182

Sardinia, 130–131

saturated fats, 32, 63–64, 69–70, 252. See also fats

SCORE2 (Systematic Coronary Risk Evaluation 2), 106

screen time, sleep and, 127

screening, 14

seafood, 88, 178, 263–264

secondary prevention
  defined, 14, 109
  goal of, 158, 159
  medications as, 150–152
  overview of, 99–103
  statins for, 150, 151, 152
sedentary lifestyle, 32
seeds, 88, 178, 197, 261–262
selenium, 75
self-care, 124–125, 168, 256–257
serotonin, 143, 144
sesame seeds, 262
Seven Countries Study, 40, 87
seven-day meal plan, 203–208
sexual health, 86
side effects, 116, 161
Simon Poole's Positively Good For You Heart, 214
simvastatin, 14
sitosterolemia, 31, 157
sleep, 34–35, 50, 51, 126–129, 256
small plate recipes, 221–227
smoking, 10, 13, 35, 53, 124
social connection, 129–131
socioeconomic factors, 113–114
soda, 62, 66
sofrito, 93
soluble fiber, 72
Spiced Quinoa and Lentil Sliders recipe, 223
Spinach, Lentil, and Pomegranate Salad
    recipe, 238
spiritual meditation, 142
stanols, 73, 157
statin complacency, 13
statins
  benefits of, 102–103, 115, 116–117, 151, 272
  conflicts of interest regarding, 104
  defined, 102
  drug interactions with, 160
  evidence from, 104
  function of, 14, 102, 114, 151

  importance of, 14
  inflammation and, 102–103
  myth regarding, 272
  needed to harm (NNH) and, 119
  needed to treat (NNT) and, 119
  overview of, 154
  oxidation and, 103
  plaque and, 103
  primary prevention, 116
  publication bias and, 104
  recommendations for, 104
  risk reduction from, 110, 158–159
  as secondary prevention, 150, 151, 152
  side effects of, 103, 115, 116–117, 154
  statistics regarding, 271
  stopping/starting, 115–118
  talking to doctor about, 118–119
stearic acid, 64, 71
sterols, 18, 73, 157
stress/chronic stress
  breathwork for, 141–142
  high cholesterol and, 34–35
  hormones and, 256
  inflammation and, 53
  managing, 139–144
  mindfulness for, 142–143
  oxidative stress and, 50
  reducing, 137–145
  as risk factor, 125, 133
  yoga for, 140–141
stroke (cerebrovascular accident), 12, 43,
    55–56, 162
students, stress and, 138
subendothelial space, 41
substance use disorder, 124
sugar, myth regarding, 273–274
supplements, 127–128, 170
surgery, 162–163
Sweet Cardamom-Scented Barley and Strawberry
    Pudding with Nuts recipe, 219

sympathetic nervous system, 124
synapses, 19

T

tapping, 169
TC/HDL ratio, 25
tea, 92, 170
tendinous xanthomas, 31
terminal illness, 117
testosterone, 18
thromboembolism, 54
thrombus (blood clot), 44, 45, 54, 57, 103, 269
thyroid disorders, 36
thyroxine, 36
Tomato Basil Sauce recipe, 183
total cholesterol (TC) level, 21, 23, 25
toxins, 50
trans fats, 32, 62–63, 179, 252
transcendental meditation, 143
transient ischemic attack (TIA), 41, 55, 150
treatment. *See also* medications, cholesterol-lowering
  future research and developments in, 161
  medication considerations in, 150–153
  monitoring, 161
  overview of, 149
  personalizing, 157–161
  primary prevention, 99–103, 116, 152–153, 158, 159
  secondary prevention, 14, 100, 109, 151, 152, 158, 159
  surgical interventions for, 162–163
  survey of medications for, 153–157
  targets and dosing in, 158–159
triglycerides (TGs)
  categorization of levels of, 24
  defined, 20
  in foods, 64
  high levels of, 26
  measurement of, 21

medications for, 155
omega-3 fatty acids for, 157
taming, 26
type 2 diabetes and, 33
variability in, 24, 25
type 2 diabetes, 33, 57, 83, 152

U

ultra-processed foods (UPFs), 32, 62, 65–67, 200
ultrasound, 46
ultraviolet radiation (UV), 49
unsaturated fats, 32, 63, 73. *See also* fats

V

vascular diseases, 12, 13. *See also* cardiovascular diseases (CVDs)
vascular pathology, 8
vascular system, 9
vasodilators, 163
Vegetable Stir-Fry with Edamame and Brown Rice Noodles recipe, 232
vegetables, 88, 92, 177–179, 265. *See also* Mediterranean diet/lifestyle
veins, 9
very low-density lipoprotein (VLDL), 20, 26, 155
very low-density lipoprotein (VLDL-C) component, 33
Virchow, Rudolf, 11
visceral fat, 33
vitamin C, 74
vitamin D, 19, 75
vitamin E, 74
vitamins, 18, 19, 74–75

W

Walk at Home, 137
websites
  Amy Riolo Selections Extra Virgin Olive Oil, 214
  Atherosclerotic Cardiovascular Disease (ASCVD) Risk Estimator, 105

websites *(continued)*
  Brad Yates, 169
  Calm, 124
  community-supported agriculture (CSA), 176
  Headspace, 124, 142
  Monterey Bay Aquarium, 264
  QRISK Risk Calculator, 106
  Simon Poole's Positively Good For You
    Heart, 214
  Walk at Home, 137
  Yoga with Adriene, 141
  YouTube, 137
weight gain, high cholesterol and, 32, 33
Western diet, 82–85, 94
white coat effect, 113
whole grains, 87, 178, 197, 264
whole wheat, 264
World Health Organization (WHO), 7, 23, 63, 136

X

xanthelasma, 31

Y

Yates, Brad, 169
yoga, 140–141
Yoga with Adriene, 141
yogurt, 264–265
YouTube, 137
Yuka, 67

Z

Za'atar Spiced Pita Chips recipe, 191
zinc, 75

About the Authors

Simon Poole, MD: Simon has been a primary care physician in Cambridge, England, for more than 30 years with a particular interest in public health, lifestyle medicine, and nutrition, as well as the management of long-term medical conditions. He has taught and undertaken research with Cambridge University and is a founding member of the British and European Associations of Lifestyle Medicine. Simon is a council member of the U.S. True Health Initiative and an International Senior Collaborator with the Global Centre for Nutrition and Health in Cambridge. He was awarded Fellowship of the British Medical Association for services to the profession in 2018, which included long-standing membership in the Council of the Royal College of General Practitioners and Public Health Medicine Committee. Simon is a recognized international authority and speaker on lifestyle medicine, chairing the Food Values Conference series at the Pontifical Academy of Science of the Vatican, and the author of the award-winning book *The Olive Oil Diet* (Hachette), *The Real Mediterranean Diet* (Cambridge Academic), and *Olive Oil For Dummies* and the latest editions of *Diabetes For Dummies, Diabetes Meal Planning & Nutrition For Dummies,* and the *Diabetes Cookbook For Dummies* (all published by John Wiley & Sons) with Amy Riolo.

Amy Riolo: Amy Riolo is a best-selling author and an award-winning chef, television host, and Mediterranean diet ambassador. The author of 20 books (this book is the 21st), she has been named Knight of the Order of the Star of Italy by the Italian government; "The Ambassador of Italian Cuisine in the U.S." by the Italian International Agency for Foreign Press; "Ambassador of the Italian Mediterranean Diet" by the International Academy of the Italian Mediterranean Diet in her ancestral homeland of Calabria, Italy; and "Ambassador of Mediterranean Cuisine in the World" by the Rome-based media agency *We The Italians.* In 2019, she launched her own private-label collection of premium Italian imported culinary ingredients called Amy Riolo Selections, which includes extra-virgin olive oil, balsamic vinegar, and pesto sauce from award-winning artisan companies.

Dedication

Simon Poole: I dedicate my contributions to this book to Tahmineh Zamani Ranjbar.

Amy Riolo: I dedicate my contributions to this book to my father, Rick Riolo, for inspiring me to cook and become a culinary anthropologist, and for his overwhelming support.

Authors' Acknowledgments

The authors want to thank Tracy Boggier for being so enthusiastic, efficient, and great to work with. We truly appreciate the expert and efficient editorial support and guidance of Elizabeth Kuball and thank Kristie Pyles for all of her support as well. Many thanks to Rachel Nix for her meticulous recipe testing and nutritional analysis.

Cholesterol science is expanding all the time and is not without controversies — we would not embark on a project like this without having confidence in a technical editor who brings experience, knowledge, and wisdom; we would like to thank Dr. Gabriele Mocciaro for his support. We're very fortunate to have had his guidance throughout the writing of the book.

Dr. Simon Poole: It has been a great honor for me to write another book in the *For Dummies* series with Amy, who is a constant source of inspiration and whose alchemy turns medical facts and figures into practical and delicious recipes for life. I would also like to thank my family and friends who are so supportive in all my endeavors.

Throughout my life, I have been profoundly fortunate to study and work in environments where new evidence is met with curiosity, explored through research, integrated into practice, and, when necessary, questioned with thoughtful critique. This journey began in my childhood in the university town of Aberystwyth, Wales, and continued through my medical studies in London, my clinical practice and public health work in Cambridge, and my engagement with the British Medical Association. I am deeply grateful to the colleagues and mentors, past and present, who embody a commitment to lifelong learning. They have shown me the value of approaching contentious topics with both passion and open-mindedness, and where disagreements arise, responding with patience, courtesy, and compassion. My patients, too, have been among my greatest teachers, imparting invaluable lessons about the importance of respectful listening, shared and informed decision-making, and recognizing individual values and preferences. Their experiences have also reinforced the need to challenge traditional, paternalistic models of medical care. If *Managing Cholesterol For Dummies* offers readers a fresh understanding grounded in these principles, it will be a testament to the many individuals who have shaped my thinking. I remain profoundly indebted to all those who have taught me, and continue to teach me, the enduring importance of curiosity, humility, and empathy in medicine and beyond.

Amy Riolo: My earliest memories of cooking were with my mother, Faith Riolo, who taught me that food was not just something we eat to nourish ourselves, but an edible gift that could be given to express love. When she was later diagnosed with diabetes, it was my love for her and desire to create delicious and nutritious meals for my parents that eventually led me to write books on wellness. I owe much of my professional culinary success to my father, Rick Riolo, for always believing in my talent and supporting my career goals. To my beloved little brother, Jeremy — you are my why, and I'm grateful to be able to pass our family's knowledge down to you.

My Nonna, Angela Magnone Foti, taught me to cook and bake, as well as valuable lessons that served me outside of the kitchen. My Yia Yia, Mary Michos Riolo, shared her beloved Greek traditions with me as well. I would probably never have published a cookbook if it weren't for my mentor, Sheilah Kaufman, who patiently taught me much more than I ever planned on learning. I'm proud to pass her knowledge on to others. Without the assistance and guidance of my late friend, spirit sister, and healer Kathleen Ammalee Rogers, I'd never have been able to realize my professional writing goals. I'm very thankful to Chef Luigi Diotaiuti, for always believing in me and for encouraging me to foster my dreams and goals.

There are dozens of people whom I'm proud to call friends and colleagues and interact with daily, each of whom indirectly enable me to achieve my goals. I'm grateful to each of you. I would like to thank Italian President Mattarella, Minsistro Gonzalez of the Embassy of Italy in the United States, and Counselor Michela Carboniero of the Italian Cultural Institute for giving me the honor of being titled Knight of the Order of the Star of Italy. I would also like to thank my dear friends and importers of Amy Riolo Selections products, Stefano and Davide Ferrari, for distributing them. Many thanks to all of my wonderful producers — Tenute Cristiano, Olio Anfosso, Pasta Marella, and Acetaia Castelli for their partnerships. In Calabria, Italy, I would like to thank my cousins, Angela Riolo, Pina and Franco Riolo, Tonia Riolo, and Mario Riolo for increasing my knowledge and for their support. I would also like to thank chefs Salvatore Murano and Enzo Murano of Max Trattoria Enoteca for including me in their culinary-cultural pursuits in Italy and for naming me an honorary member of Associazione Regionale Cuochi Pittagorici (ARCP). I am very grateful to the Italian Trade Agency in New York and the Embassy of Italy in Washington, D.C., for the opportunities and honors that they have bestowed upon me. *Mille grazie* to Dr. Battista Liserre for his inspirational work on nourishing both the mind and the soul, and to Silvestro Parise for including me in projects that promote Calabria. To my dear friends Jonathan Bardzik, Gail Broeckel, Ann Hotung, Sharon Wolpoff, Jeff Fritz, Paul Kolze, Stu Hershey, Maria Fusco, and Kim Foley, you're my spirit family and I'm blessed to have you in my life. Many thanks to Melissa's Produce for their generous donation of produce for recipe development. Many thanks to my tour partner, Alex Safos of Indigo Gazelle Tours, for the fantastic opportunities to cook and write in Morocco and Greece. And finally, I would like to thank my coauthor, Dr. Simon Poole, for his tremendous knowledge and commitment to the cause of promoting health and happiness, for always inspiring me, and for valuing my voice. It's a pleasure and an honor to collaborate with you.

Publisher's Acknowledgments

Managing Editor: Murari Mukundan

Executive Editor: Tracy Boggier

Editor: Elizabeth Kuball

Technical Editor: Gabriele Mocciaro, PhD

Production Editor: Bharaneedharan Murthy

Recipe Tester: Rachel Nix

Nutrition Analysis: Rachel Nix

Cover Image: © fcafotodigital/Getty Images

Special Help: Carmen Krikorian, Kristie Pyles

12 301